Comme

"A compassionate and heart warming story of one woman's struggle to find answers to a disease that few knew anything about. It shares real life experiences and an abundance of tips for day-to-day, caregiving practices that help us survive the struggle of Alzheimer's disease.

"This book is a **must** for families, support groups, and caregiving staff alike."

> Pat Warner, RN, MSN
> Director, Curry Manor

"Compelling, informative & touching. Well written. "

> Barbara Gillogly, Ph. D.
> Coordinator, Gerontology Program
> American River College
> Sacramento, California

"...a compelling story of personal courage, determination, and faith triumphing over adversity."

> Helen Davies, RN, MS, RNCS
> Stanford Alzheimer's Center
> Stanford Univ. School of Medicine
> Palo Alto, California

"A courageous, bittersweet story of one woman's experience, first as a young child, Alzheimer's caregiver of her mother, to witnessing her siblings being afflicted one by one.

"The love that came into her life as a young woman has been her anchor in the storm of pain produced by Alzheimer's disease.

Comments from experts

"This is a tale of love and faith that made it possible for her to survive the challenges faced by over four million Americans today.

"This book gives its readers direct insights into the stages of the disease with honest reality. It is an important addition to the growing literature on the crisis at our door."

Joy Glenner, President, CEO
The George G. Glenner
Alzheimer's Family Centers, Inc.
San Diego, California

"No one knows the depth of pain of Alzheimer's disease except those who have experienced it. We in the scientific community must never lose our human touch in the name of objectivity. People become ill. Family members suffer. Loss is profound. It does hurt. It hurts to get close, even as researchers. We would like to pull back and ignore the anguish. But we must embrace it as we hug the family members, for we really are connected one to another.

"The disease robs us of so much. It must not be allowed to rob us of our empathy. Bea Gorman's life story, WILL I BE NEXT?, written by Lois Bristow, brings us closer to the pain, the reality, and also to the courage, hope, love, and humanness of those suffering with Alzheimer's disease in their families."

Gary D. Miner, Ph.D.
Linda A. Winters-Miner, Ph.D.
The Alzheimer's Foundation
Familial Alzheimer's Disease
Research Foundation
Southern Nazarene University
Tulsa, Oklahoma

Comments from experts

"Not often, but now and then folks get a chance to read a story that can touch the hearts at the deepest level. Bea Gorman's life does just that. She is an inspiration to all who hope to face life's challenges with courage and faith. To read her life story is to take a quiet walk with a proud and sweet lady."

Randall W. Rosa', Attorney at Law
National Academy of Elder Law Attorneys
Sacramento, California

WILL I BE NEXT? is an inspiring account of a woman turning painful experience into meaningful life as Alzheimer's disease cut a deadly swath through her family.

"This book also provides a compendium of useful tips about how to care for someone with Alzheimer's disease. The simple way these ideas have been laid out is appealing, appropriatively tentative, and easy to read and try."

Robert Cook-Deegan, M.D.
National Academy of Sciences

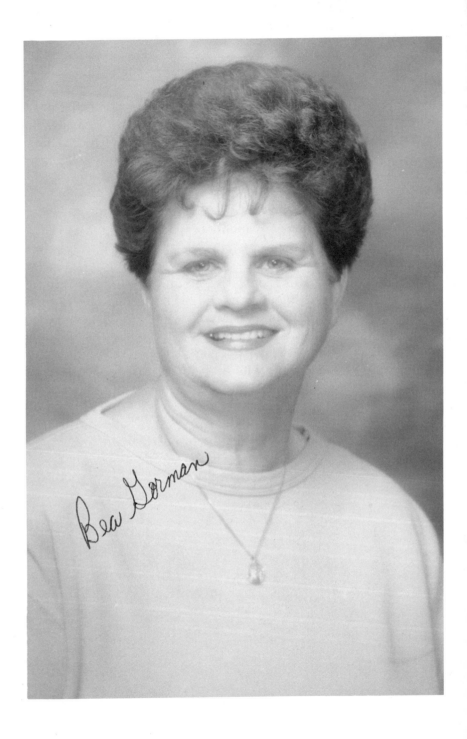

Bea Gorman

Will I Be Next?

The Terror of Living with Familial Alzheimer's Disease

Bea Gorman's Life Story

by Lois Bristow

HopeWarren Press   Acampo, California

HopeWarren Press
P.O. Box 204
Acampo, CA 95220

© 1996 by Lois Bristow and Bea Gorman

ISBN: 0-9648885-0-5
Library of Congress Catalog Card Number 95-80813

First edition, first printing

Layout & production by DIMI PRESS
Cover art by Sheila Somerville
Cover design by Bruce DeRoos
Printing by Gilliland Printing, Inc.

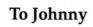

To Johnny

FOREWORD

Five members of Bea Gorman's family were struck by Alzheimer's disease. The age of onset is quite predictable in the early forties and fits the dominant-gene model of inheritance. Bea Gorman's story is an inspiring demonstration of how one person can make a tremendous impact on our world. Her story is a remarkable account, not of only coping with difficulty, but of endeavoring to make things different for others .

Bea Gorman has been the recipient of many awards over the past ten years, including the Jefferson Award, for outstanding public service. The Gormans have been influential in the California state assembly and have worked with the Governor's Task Force on Alzheimer's Disease.

Additionally, Bea and her husband, John, have served on the advisory board of the University of California, Davis, Alzheimer's Disease Center.

On February 19,1987, Mrs. Gorman was featured on the CBS Evening News with Dan Rather, along with Dr. James Gusella (Harvard) and Dr. Michael Conneally (University of Indiana Medical Center) at the first public announcement of the discoveries of "gene markers" for the FAD (Familial Alzheimer's Disease) gene and the amyloid gene. Today, summer 1995, two genes for the early onset FAD have been discovered.

These genes will prove to be the most important discoveries about Alzheimer's disease and will lead to the development of early diagnostic tests and effective treatments, and hopefully a cure.

Bea Gorman's pioneering spirit and willingness to cooperate in every way in the study of FAD has been of invaluable help to researchers in their quest to understand Alzheimer's disease. Her efforts also resulted in the establishment of support groups throughout Central and Northern California. Over the years, Bea and her husband John have spoken almost daily to service clubs, community groups, and nursing homes, providing in-service training to the staff members.

Our lives have been enriched tremendously by having known and worked with the Gormans. We have traveled up and down the State of California, testing members of Bea's family, with our "headquarters" being the Gorman home in Lodi. Their door was always open, even at 2:00 a.m., when we would quietly slip in after a lengthy day of testing and a long drive from Fresno or wherever.

The life events and circumstances that shaped Bea Gorman into what she is today are told in this book. We had difficulty putting it down. We hope you will enjoy it as much as we did and find your life enriched for having shared in her life.

Gary Miner, Ph.D. and Linda Winters-Miner, Ph.D.

The Alzheimer's Foundation (Familial Alzheimer's Disease Research Foundation) and Southern Nazarene University, Tulsa, Oklahoma. (August, 1995)

CONTENTS

INTRODUCTION

Will I Be Next? is essentially two books in one. Book One, "Bea's Story," is an inspiring account of a woman turning painful experience into meaningful life. It is, in a sense, a story of devastation and the spiritual triumph of its refugees over a foe that remains to be conquered.

Although Alzheimer's disease is rampant, the early-onset, familial Alzheimer's disease that struck the King family is comparatively rare. This book vividly tells what it means to be living with Alzheimer's disease in specific, highly relevant terms. Although it is the story of an extreme form of a very common disease, the manifestation of symptoms are the same.

For those who have been through the war of caring for someone with Alzheimer's disease, Book One offers comfort and inspiration.

Book Two, "Help for The Caregiver", is a compendium of useful tips about how to care for someone with dementia, sharing tricks of the trade accumulated over the years—no one of which works consistently, all of which have worked at one time or other, and many of which have worked in a variety of cases. The simple way they have been laid out is appealing, appropriately tentative, and easy to read and try. For those in the throes of caring for an Alzheimer's victim, it offers practical ideas for lightening the load.

For those just entering the terrifying world of becoming a caregiver to a person with Alzheimer's disease, Book Two will provide practical support and guidance. There is reassurance in knowing you are not alone and in understanding what you can expect. It is in the early stages that decisions are most crucial and good information is most useful. Book Two offers clear, practical ideas, points out decisions to be faced, and tells where a caregiver can turn for help.

Robert Cook-Deegan, M.D.
National Academy of Sciences
Washington D. C.
September, 1995

Family of Susie Hales King

Bold : Victims of Alzheimer's disease

Parents unknown

Parents died 1878 (flu epidemic)

Minnie Warren Hayles* 1872-1899 (childbirth) — John Franklin Hayles* 1867-1942

Harmon 1894-1953 (died in fire)

Susie 1896-1948

Amy 1898-1985

Frank** 1901-unk.

Corinne** 1903

John Henry** 1906-1932 (accident)

Minnie Kate** 1909-1939 (childbirth)

Dorothy Ruth** 1913

Ruth 1916-1984 (heart)

Herschel 1918-1972

Minnie Sue 1921-1974

Mary 1923

Tommy Lou 1925

Leonard 1928-1982

Norma Jean 1930-1992

Anna June 1933

Bea 1935

*name later changed to Hales

** half brothers and sisters

Five Oldest Children of Susie King

Bold: Victims of Alzheimer's disease

Four Youngest Children of Susie King

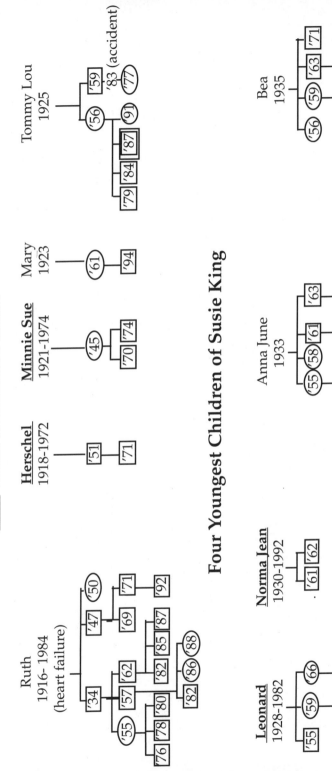

BOOK ONE

Bea's Story

CHAPTER ONE

April, 1948

The snow had melted, leaving the earth bare and ugly. Mud from our yard and the street gutters clung to anything it touched. It was April, and only the stingiest hint of green promised that spring would come. Within weeks, lush leaves would be everywhere. But when my mother died, spring was not yet here, and the neighborhood stood barren and leafless.

My mother died on April 5, 1948, shortly after my thirteenth birthday. I remember hearing people speak of her as the beauty of the family. Mama was shy and unassuming. She was also very sweet. Everyone talked about how sweet my mother was. I remember them describing her smile and her laughter revealing perfect teeth, straight, white, and glistening.

The mother I knew had no teeth. Nor did she smile. There was no laughter when I knew her. My mother lay in sullen silence. Helpless and mute.

Our family was poor, and the poor took care of their own. No one even considered having nursing help or sending Mama to a nursing home. The family took care of her. There were four of us kids still at home, and we each did our share. Daddy bathed her. My older sisters changed her bedding, including the soiled padding beneath her. Ruth, the oldest, made her night gowns. She and my other sisters dressed her and fed her, turning her often in a futile attempt to prevent bed sores. They cleaned her room and opened the windows to air out the heavy smell of sickness. For almost two years, from the time I was eleven until Mama died, it was my job to feed her lunch everyday.

During that entire time, Mama never spoke to me. Not once in all the times I fed her. I would go into her room, hoping this would be the day. I fantasized hearing her soft voice saying, "Hello, Bea," or, "I love you," or, "How are you, Bea?" or maybe she would say, "Thank you for bringing me lunch." I was always so sure this would be the day, but it never was.

Once she said quite clearly, "What's the matter?" but she hadn't said it to me. Her words just floated about the room, detached and not part of any conversation.

Although she never spoke, she watched me. Always. Her eyes, dark and dull, stuck to me like metal filings to a magnet. Her stare had a kind of disconnected, passive intensity. No recognition. No response. She just held me in the grip of her eyes.

I longed to have a mother like the mothers of my friends. Their mothers fixed their suppers and sewed their dresses, braided their hair and laughed, and loved them, and yes, scolded them. I wanted a mother who baked cookies. My friend's mother would say, "How's Mama's Angel Girl?" I knew that my mother would never call me her "Angel Girl." My mother didn't speak to me. I would have loved it if she just would have said my name.

Of her nine children, I was the youngest, her baby child. I remember her rocking me before she was bed-ridden, crooning her favorite song, "Jesus Loves Me, This I Know." I was much too big to be rocked like a baby, and my feet dragged back and forth on the floor, but it didn't matter. Hungry to be held and nestled in the warmth of her arms, I was lulled by her singing and soothed by the rhythmic creak of the rocking chair. Today, I cherish rocking my grandchildren and singing to them as my mother sang to me. I hope that some-day, when I am gone, they will look back and remember the warmth and the love we shared.

For as long as I can remember, I never had the mother I longed to have. Instead, in some skewed way, I was the parent, an unmothered waif, clothes un-matched and disheveled, straight blonde hair un-combed, large, hazel-green eyes sad and resentful. It was my job to take care of her. It was not her job to take care of me.

Each day I fed her lunch. The job was tedious and slow. Mama never responded. She was a non-per-son who didn't know me. She was never hungry, and I, without patience, forced spoonful after spoonful into my reluctant, disinterested, unappreciative patient, scooping rejected food from her face and chin and shov-ing it back into her resisting mouth. Often an hour or more would go by, and most of her meal would remain uneaten and cold.

I remember so clearly one noontime in early summer. As usual, I was feeding my lifeless mother. It was a light and inviting day, before the stifling humidity arrived to suffocate everything and everyone. Through the open window came the sounds of my friends playing. Laughter and chatter filled the world just beyond our front porch door. I was not yet twelve, and I ached to be with them.

Feeding progress was unusually slow. I tried to force another spoonful and failed. To speed things up, I sneaked a few bites and then a few more. Soon my task was finished, and I was free to join the play. Taking a few bites to speed up the task of feeding worked so well that I used the same technique again.

When Mama stopped eating completely and her seizures increased, Daddy knew it was a matter of time until she died, and he didn't want us kids to be alone with her when she passed away. He told us that it was best to put her in the county home. Mama died three weeks later.

At her funeral, I overheard two women talking about her death, saying that she had died of malnutrition, that she "had literally starved to death, poor woman." I might as well have been struck by lightning. My newly-turned-thirteen-year-old conscience responded with overpowering guilt, for I knew then with absolute clarity that I was responsible. I pretended not to hear the women talking and vowed never to breathe a word to anyone that my mama was dead because I didn't feed her right. No one must ever know that I, however unwittingly, had killed my own mother.

Thirty-six years later, at the funeral of my sister Ruth, I was talking to a relative by marriage who had known me as a child. She mentioned how impressed she had been with how our family had all pitched in to help take care of my mama and how, at such a young age, I had done my share. She told me of a time when she had been in our upstairs bedroom when I was feeding Mama.

My heart stopped. This woman knew. Fearing the worst, I was somehow compelled to ask. "Did I feed her all of it? Her meal. You know, did I feed her everything on her plate?"

My question was hesitant. Dreading the answer, I felt my breath catch in my throat as I waited for her response.

"Oh, yes, everything. You fed her everything. You did such a wonderful job." She smiled warmly. "I have always admired the way you took care of your dear, sweet mama."

It was an off-handed, innocent response from a person whom I had not seen in over thirty years and probably would never see again, but the cloud was lifted, and the haunting guilt I had carried since childhood was finally gone.

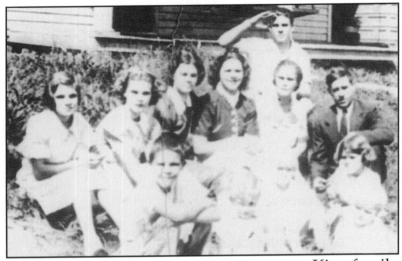

King family

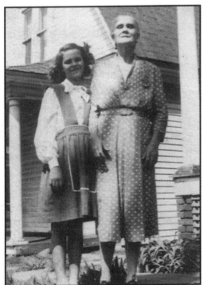

Bea and mother

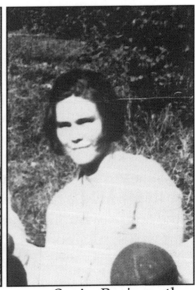

Susie, Bea's mother

CHAPTER TWO

Childhood

When my mother died, very little was known about Alzheimer's disease. "Pre-senile dementia" was listed on her death certificate. She had died from the effects of pre-senile dementia. Basically, they said that she had lost her mind early in life. We knew that, but we had no idea that others were going through this same horrifying nightmare. We knew that something was terribly wrong with her, and that she couldn't do even the simplest, everyday things that normal people can do. We also knew that something had gone wrong with the spinal test they had done at the hospital, but we didn't know that she had a disease. She came home from the hospital totally helpless, so we took care of her. That's what a family does, takes care of someone in the family who is sick. After all, she was our mama.

If what happened to Mama had happened today, somebody would have been held accountable, but the mistake was made a long time ago on the mother of a poor and unsophisticated family. A mistake was

made, and my mama, permanently silenced and paralyzed, was sent home to die.

Years later, Mama's oldest son would be the first
of four of her nine children to fall prey to the same
disease. Herschel died in 1972. He was fifty-four years
old. The doctor's acknowledged that he died from the
effects of Alzheimer's disease, but in 1972, there was
nowhere for his family to turn for help. For years
Herschel's erratic and irrational behavior, his angry
rages, and his inability to hold a job left his wife and
son confused and often desperate, helpless to do anything for Herschel or for themselves.

Two years after Herschel died, and just two
months shy of her fifty-fourth birthday, my sister
Minnie Sue passed away, dead from the effects of
Alzheimer's disease. She had suffered for years as the
disease ate away at her mind, leaving her unable to
work, and finally, unable to function.

My brother Leonard, ten years younger than
Herschel, began showing symptoms. His family
thought he'd gone off the deep end. His irrational and
unruly conduct cost him his marriage because his wife
and son had no idea that he was doing all these strange
things because he was a sick man. They only knew that
the things he did couldn't be tolerated. He died in 1982,
ten years after his older brother died. He, too, was fifty-
four. He died from the effects of Alzheimer's disease,
but for most of those years when he was doing all those
crazy things, no one told his family what the problem
was.

Norma Jean, two years younger than Leonard, was behaving strangely. She, too, was doing peculiar things. Nobody in our family wanted to admit that she might be in the throes of dementia. My sister Norma Jean died in 1992 from the effects of Alzheimer's disease.

Doctors told us that Alzheimer's disease was rare. They also said that it almost never ran in families.

I'm telling my story, hoping to help others. Hundreds of thousands have been struck with this treacherous killer. Their families have been decimated. When a loved one suffers, the family suffers, too. I think the families are as much the victims as the ones who are actually sick. They pay emotionally, financially, and physically. Pain, grief, anger, and guilt come hand in hand, in partnership with this plague.

If I had known then what I know now, my life would have been less terrifying. If sharing my story can help even a few, if it can lighten the load and lessen pain, if the feeling of isolation can be eased by knowing where to turn for help, this book will have been worthwhile.

For years, the doctors told me that my chances of becoming ill with Alzheimer's disease were fifty-fifty. I decided to gamble on the winning fifty percent and dedicate my life to helping those who are the caregivers of Alzheimer's patients.

In the beginning, as I spoke to various groups, I always saw myself as someday being the victim of

Alzheimer's disease. As I described what happened to my mama and brothers and sisters, I knew that I was describing what was going to happen to me. Burdened by this fear, I would not have been able to continue without my abiding faith in God and my absolute certainty that, whatever happened to me, God would always be with me.

As far back as I can remember, Alzheimer's disease, even though at the time I didn't know the word and didn't know it was a disease, clouded my childhood. I have forgotten many things about growing up, but of the things I do remember, the joys and pains remain with me as though the experiences had happened yesterday.

Mama and Daddy married in 1915, when she was nineteen, and he was twenty-one. Over the next twenty years, nine children were born to this union. In spite of our chaotic childhood, all nine of us turned out to be responsible, hard working adults, at least, until the disease struck.

Ruth, their first child born, arrived almost a year to the day after my parent's wedding. Herschel arrived two years later, followed by Minnie Sue, Mary, Tommy Lou, Leonard, Norma Jean, and Anna June. Finally, on March 23, 1935, I came along. Mama was thirty-nine years old. My mama, Herschel, Minnie Sue, Leonard, and Norma Jean were all victims of Alzheimer's disease. I've always found it strange that both of my brothers died from the disease, and each sister born after a brother also died from the disease.

My older brothers and sisters remember Mama when she was normal. Mama's loving care played a big role in influencing her children. By her example, she was the one who taught us responsibility. Mama taught us values. The older kids remember her cleaning and washing and cooking, singing lullabies, doing all of the mother-kind-of things that mothers do. I don't remember her doing any of that. They reminisced about her scrumptious blueberry cobblers, her out-of-this-world carrot cakes, and her delicious, simple southern cooking. I don't remember Mama cooking at all. For as long as I can remember, she didn't cook, or clean house, or do laundry, or garden. Most of the time she sat at the head of the stairs reading her Bible, or staring blankly, or slumped over sound asleep. My daddy would be furious when he came home hungry and tired to find his meals not ready and his clothes neither washed nor ironed. Nobody realized how sick Mama really was.

I do remember one time when my mama was there for me, though. I had an argument with my closest friend, Gloria Howard, and ran home crying. Mama came back to the Howard's house with me and helped me retrieve my belongings that Gloria wouldn't let me have. I have always treasured that act, reminding myself that I did have a mother when I needed one, and knowing that if she wasn't sick, she really would do things for me because she really did care.

In the beginning, when Mama first began to forget things and act strangely, people couldn't understand what was wrong with her. They had no idea she was sick. For awhile they wondered if having so many children caused her problems. Later, when it was clear to everyone that she was really very ill, Daddy felt bad because he had been so mad at her for not doing what she was supposed to do.

She was in bad shape when Daddy finally took her to the hospital for tests. On the way in, the last thing I remember my mama saying was, "I hope they find out what's wrong with me." They didn't. My mother walked into the hospital and was carried out on a stretcher and brought home in an ambulance. They had given her a spinal tap and something had gone wrong. She neither walked nor talked again. Never again did she read her beloved Bible. She just lay in her bed and stared. Daddy would sometimes sit her up in her rocker. She would sit and stare.

I thought at the time that the mistake they made at the hospital was the worst thing that could ever have happened to her, but after I had seen my brothers and sisters go through the slow, horrifying, debilitating stages of the disease, I think perhaps that mistake was a blessing in disguise. My mother didn't have to suffer through all of the agonizing stages of this cruel, vicious killer called Alzheimer's disease.

Mama's long, thick, dark hair came below her waist. Had it been any longer she would have sat on it. She wore it in braids as round as my wrists. When she was bedridden, Daddy cut her hair. It was too much trouble to take care of. He just chopped it off. To me, cutting her hair was a violation of her dignity. More of a violation even than seeing my sisters change her nightgown. Mama had always been extremely modest. It was a shock to me to see my mother's naked body, but it was seeing her hair cut short that always made me sad.

I remember the house where I grew up, a two-story, wood-sided structure, painted white, located on a street with similar, nondescript houses in a poor neighborhood. Our address was 908 Reynolds Street, which was about one third of the way up from the bottom of the hill. Reynolds Street was a cobbled road that ran east and west between two hills, down into a ravine and up again. It was a challenge getting up either side in the winter when roads were slick with ice, and a person couldn't go anywhere without going up one of those hills.

Our small front porch served as a gathering place. The lattice work below the porch provided a foundation, and the posts of the porch framed the setting where so many significant events in my life took place. I sat on that porch as a small child and as a teenager, and with Johnny in the early days of our courtship. I remember the two of us sitting in the porch swing, our silly chatter and my giggling. Johnny and I married while we were still in our teens.

Before Mama was confined to bed, I stood with her in front of that porch, and Daddy took our picture. It is the only picture I have of me with Mama. After Mama's funeral, pictures of all the people who came were taken on that porch. I sat on that porch swing as a bride, my white gown spread out around me. In a myriad of ways, what took place on our front porch summarized my childhood.

As a child I thought of our house as large, and I always felt that, although we were poor, we were also somewhat privileged because we had an indoor bathroom while many of our neighbors still used out houses. I remember the stairway as a retreat of sorts. I would pull the phone cord tightly around the corner and close the door as far as I could to take private phone calls from teenage friends. I talked to Johnny a lot from that stairway.

Many years later, Johnny and I went back to see that house in Kansas City, Kansas, and I was shocked to see how small it was and amazed that a family of eleven could have survived there. But we did.

Of course, Ruth was married before I was born, so I guess ten were all that lived there at one time. By the time I was five, Herschel had gone off to war, and Minnie Sue had married and left home. Still, it was hard to comprehend a big family living in that house without bursting the seams.

The downstairs consisted of a foyer, which barely held a library table and fold-away-couch where my two brothers slept, the front room, dining room, and kitchen. The phone was on that library table next to the stairway. All rooms were small. Upstairs were two bedrooms. One struggled to hold two double beds, one where my daddy and mama slept and the other for Anna June, Norma Jean and me. There was hardly any room left for us to squeeze past the beds. The front bedroom was across a narrow hall. The two older girls, Mary and Tommy Lou, slept there. There was a tiny bathroom at the head of the stairs between the bedrooms, and a closet that Leonard used as a special hideaway.

My oldest sister Ruth married before I was born. She and her husband Joe lived one block away from our house on Reynolds Street. Ruth was like a mother to me. I remember going to her house at supper time when she always had a meal ready for her family. Meals weren't ready at our house.

Ruth's oldest child Sonny and I are almost the same age, and in many ways, he was more like a brother to me than my own brothers. We were always together. I remember he had a paper route, and I would ride on the handle bars of his bike when he delivered papers. When we wanted to go to the movie show, we would make the rounds of his paper route and collect just enough cash, fourteen cents to be exact, to buy two tickets to the local theater, and off we would go to a movie. The rest of the collections would have to wait. Sonny and I had great times together.

By the time I could remember Ruth, Herschel and Minnie Sue, they were all adults living their own lives. I remember Mary and Tommy Lou, though, primping and getting dressed up all fancy to go to the USO to dance with the soldiers and sailors. It was a patriotic duty they enjoyed immensely. I thought of them as being so very sophisticated and dreamed of the day when I would be grown up and could go to such places and dance with boys.

Mary and Tommy Lou left Kansas City and went to Hollywood. Both women were beautiful, but more than that, they both had a sophisticated, polished air about them. They had glamour. Both knew how to do their makeup and hair and how to dress.

Mary was a natural blonde with flawless skin, high cheek bones, perfect features, and clear, blue eyes. When she applied for a factory job at Max Factor, she was offered a job in the makeup department instead. She had an artistic talent and soon was doing work for the movie studios. I loved to hear about her working with famous movie stars. She was very good at doing makeup and worked as a makeup artist until she retired.

Tommy Lou's ambition was to break into show business. I was enamored with the idea of having a movie star for a sister. Tommy Lou was a dark haired, green eyed beauty when she left home, but being blonde was the thing to be in Hollywood, so she became a blonde. What a beautiful blonde she was! Tommy Lou's long, shapely legs danced her right into the line of the Earl Carrol dancers, which was quite a feat for someone who had never taken dance lessons. She also landed quite a few bit parts in movies before she decided to return to Kansas.

After Mama died, eighteen-year-old Norma Jean left for Hollywood to be near her sisters and never returned to live in the Midwest.

Anna June, like our sister Mary, was blonde, blue-eyed, and pretty. She was two years older than I, and as kids, we were very close. Anna June married Leon, and they stayed in Kansas City. She and Leon had one of the happiest marriages I have ever seen. They had four kids, and their whole family was close. Anna June was a devoted homemaker. I have never seen her when she wasn't neatly dressed with her hair combed and her makeup on. Johnny reminds me often of how Anna June always catered to Leon. I remind him just as often that he didn't marry Anna June. He married me.

When Mama got sick, my daddy took care of us kids in his fashion, and I know it wasn't easy for him. He was sort of a grown-up little boy himself. But he didn't leave us, and I guess a lot of men would have. I know there were times when he would have liked to leave, but he never did. At home, we rarely had real meals where we all sat down and had dinner together. Daddy cooked mostly beans. In those days, poor people ate lots of rice and beans. We ate mostly beans. Black-eyed peas and ham hocks were always simmering on the back of the stove. My sisters would often ask what kind of beans we were having for supper. It was sort of family joke, like we were ordering an entree at a fancy restaurant.

People said Daddy was a womanizer, but as a kid, I didn't know or care about such things. My brothers knew and cared, though. That time when my mama asked, "What's the matter?", the boys and my daddy were fighting, and our poor little house shook from foundation to roof. You could hear them cursing and hitting each other and the furniture falling. My brothers didn't approve of my daddy's roving eye.

Before Mama was sick, she was the peace maker in the family. One of my older sisters told me that when things weren't "going well" at home, which usually meant that Daddy was making quite a fuss, Susie would look up at her husband in a loving way and, in her charming Southern drawl, would say, "Now, Bose, everything will be all right." They said Daddy always settled down when she did that. No one ever heard her say a harsh word to or about anyone. She was loving and gentle, except for taking the switch to us when we aggravated her.

Daddy was the rambunctious one. Mama was the steady hand. She was the disciplining hand, too, and didn't hesitate to take a willow switch to our legs and back sides when we misbehaved. Somehow, even though she didn't "spare the rod," her love for us was always there, and all of us thought of her as the gentle one. I never remember Daddy spanking or whipping any of us. He swore and talked rough and fought with the boys when they were grown, but he never whipped us.

Supporting nine children wasn't much fun, and Daddy moaned and groaned about it all the time. He had a tendency to feel sorry for himself. He may have thought the world owed him something for having all these kids, but since the world was obviously not coming through, he turned to his kids. Daddy was always after us to go to work and help him out, the sooner the better. We all started finding jobs when we were quite young. I baby-sat by the time I was ten and helped other adults clean their houses, or I'd run errands for them. I learned early to iron clothes for other people. We all did whatever we had to do to earn money since, by the time we were twelve or thirteen, we were expected to buy most of our own necessities, things like shoes and clothes.

Daddy didn't think much of education, and my brothers didn't like school and weren't the least bit interested in academics. One day Daddy was driving by Herschel's school and saw him outside picking up trash. He took Herschel out of school on the spot and put him to work. Daddy thought it wasn't right for him to be working and not be getting paid for it. I'm sure the teachers were relieved to have this high spirited, disinterested student out of their hair. Anyway, no attempt was ever made to track Herschel down and bring him back to class, or to admonish my daddy for pulling him out of school. My daddy said that he might as well work at a real job and earn some money since he wasn't learning anything at school anyway. So Herschel learned his daddy's trade and learned it well.

After Mama died, Daddy took me to his home town of Bluefield in West Virginia. I was thirteen. Anna June was not quite two years older than I, but Daddy just left her in Kansas City to fend for herself. She moved in with a family and took care of their children for awhile and then moved in with our sisters. Years

later, she told me how hurt and bitter she had been
that Daddy just up and left her there. I guess if I'd been
any older, he would have left me too, but I'm glad he
didn't.

In Bluefield, because Daddy was the baby of the
family, his sisters spoiled him rotten. I guess, after all
those years of taking care of Mama and us kids, he
was needing to be spoiled a little bit. Daddy stayed
with Bertha, his oldest sister whom we called Aunt
Bertie. I stayed with another sister, Aunt Minnie, whose
real name was Nina Mae.

The year that I lived with my Aunt Minnie in
Bluefield was the happiest and most normal year of
my childhood. I thrived. She talked to me and listened.
She offered a shoulder to cry on and a firm hand when
needed. She also gave me hugs, for which I hungered.
My Aunt Minnie saw to it that I ate three good meals a
day and wore clean clothes. Life in Bluefield was good.

It was the only year I ever did well in school.
Aunt Minnie was interested in me and in my school
work. At home, I missed school often and couldn't keep
up with the assignments. Eventually, I lost interest and
dropped out. At home, school wasn't important. In
Bluefield, school was very important, and I was encouraged to attend. My teachers found me to be an
eager student. For the first time in my life, I earned
good grades and thought school was fun.

Of course, I worked in Bluefield, too. One of my
jobs was to be a companion for an elderly woman who
was the widow of a doctor. I thought of it as a glorified

baby-sitting job. The woman was educated and refined and her house was filled with lovely things, all of which made me feel inferior and uncomfortable. The woman was nice enough, but she was cold to me, or at least, I thought she was. Part of my job was to sleep there in case she needed anything at night. The wind howled, and the trees and bushes brushed against the siding, making strange noises in a strange place. I remember feeling terribly alone and frightened. But it was a job, and I liked the I money she paid me. Actually, the money was essential, since I had to buy my own clothes and whatever else I needed.

After a year in Bluefield, we moved back to Kansas City. I hated to leave. Daddy had rented our house on Reynolds Street while we were gone because he needed the money. The renters still wanted to live there when we returned, so Daddy rented a room from them. I was shuttled off to a neighbor lady where I was supposed to work for her in exchange for renting a room. The only catch was that she didn't have a room to rent so I worked for the privilege of sleeping in her bed with her.

I stayed with this neighbor for six months and then moved in with my sisters where I lived until I graduated from the eighth grade. That was my only graduation. I went on to finish the ninth grade before I dropped out of school.

Gloria Howard was still my best friend. She was tiny, freckled, full of spunk, and definitely the leader of our twosome. I was devoted to her. We planned to live together when we grew up, and when it came time to strike out on our own, Gloria and I rented an apartment together. We had managed to earn and save enough money to rent a small place. I had just turned fifteen and was completely on my own.

CHAPTER THREE

Johnny

I was baby-sitting when I first met Johnny. At the time, he was about as round as he was tall, but he was especially nice to me. I was supposed to pick up this little girl from the St. John's Orphanage which was directly across the street from the neighborhood market. I was to take her someplace, where I can't remember, in a taxi, but I didn't have an inkling about how to call one. I asked this well mannered boy whose folks owned the grocery what I was supposed to do. He helped me get a taxi, and he's been helping me ever since.

I was ten or eleven then. Johnny and I didn't actually meet until about three years later, after Mama had died, and when I returned from that year in Bluefield. One day he was telling me that his folks used to have the grocery right across from St. John's Church. I told him that I had met a boy there once who helped me call a taxi. He said, "Hey, that was me!" I could hardly believe it. That little fat boy had grown up. He was awfully cute and no longer fat. And he was still nice to me.

One of the things that attracted me to Johnny was his family. Whenever his dad left the house, he always kissed his mother good-bye. I had never seen my daddy kiss my mother. Never. Johnny's family had a closeness that our family lacked. I craved having that kind of family closeness. I don't remember doing things as a family, except having celebrations on the 4th of July and on Christmas. We always had a tree. Twice I remember getting what I wanted for Christmas. I was thrilled. Once I wanted a desk, and I got one. A nice child's desk. Another time I received beautiful leggings and a coat just like I asked for, but most of the time, I watched my friends get the things they wanted for Christmas. At our house, we got practical things.

My brothers and sisters remember doing things as a family, but that was either before I was born or before I could remember. By the time I came along, birthdays were no big deal at our house. There's a good chance that birthdays never had been a big deal at our house. Nobody remembered anyone else's birthday because there were so many of us. Johnny's family made a big fuss about birthdays, and I loved it. They always had a cake and decorations and presents. Johnny gave me my first birthday party when I was sixteen. I'll never forget it. That party made me feel really special. I don't even remember my birthdays when I was growing up. They were just another day. Johnny made me feel important. Like being sixteen was really special. He thinks birthdays are special. It's the only day that is your very own day. Johnny and I always celebrate birthdays in our family. Today, we celebrate the birthdays of our grandchildren by doing something special with them. They can choose whatever they want to do, within reason of course. The grandkids are creative in making their choices. We've played miniature golf, been bowling and to the museum and to dinner. The grandkids choose. It's their day.

Johnny was always a go-getter while I just sort of let things happen. By the time he was eighteen, he owned a place of his own. It was a single-wide, mobile home, but it was his. We married when I was eighteen and Johnny was nineteen. We had planned to marry a year earlier, but we had a big argument over, of all things, who would be the ring bearer and flower girl at the wedding. It was such a nasty blow-up that Johnny canceled everything. I was devastated. My daddy was furious with Johnny. He knew a good thing for me when he saw it, and he didn't like the idea of Johnny leaving his little girl. But before too long, Johnny started coming around again, and in less than a year, the wedding was back on. We learned not to make a big fuss about silly, unimportant things.

We married on July 25, 1953, a year after our big break-up. This time, we didn't have any flower girls or ring bearers. Johnny's father is Croatian and his mother is German. Both are closely knit, social groups. One of the Croatian wedding customs is for the friends and family of the groom to go to the bride's house and bake this special bread for the wedding. I remember staying outside while Johnny's sisters and friends descended upon our kitchen to bake povitica, a traditional, wedding nut bread.

They busied themselves measuring and mixing vast amounts of ingredients, speaking Croatian all the while. I didn't understand a word they said, so I made myself scarce and hardly spoke to them. I didn't know what I should be doing. It was all very strange to me. Also, I was embarrassed because we didn't have a refrigerator. Ours had broken, and we didn't have the money to get it fixed or to get another one. Not having a refrigerator didn't seem to bother them at all though, and in the end, it all worked out fine.

In Croatian weddings, invitations are sent, but everyone is invited whether they receive an invitation or not. Johnny provided the food, but it was prepared by family and friends who lived in the neighborhood. For days, they cooked for our wedding reception. The Croatians made Croatian dishes, and the Germans made German dishes. We had a feast. Anna June was my maid of honor, and Gloria Howard was one of my bridesmaids. We had a wonderful wedding. I felt like a fairy princess who had found her prince.

There was no way in the world that my daddy could or would give me a wedding like that. I'm not sure if he even knew it was the normal thing to do, for the father to provide a wedding for his daughter. Anyway, Johnny gave us a wedding. He even bought me a white, satin wedding gown and veil. He arranged for the hall and flowers. Being in the food business, he was able to buy food and whiskey and beer wholesale. In addition, food was donated by suppliers. There were about a thousand people at the reception. Johnny arranged and paid for it all.

My daddy was in awe. He'd never seen anything like it. He just kept talking about the seven bartenders who dispensed ninety-one quarts of whisky and one-hundred-eighty gallons of beer. He knew the exact amount because he had asked. My daddy was really impressed.

He walked me down the aisle in a daze. Mostly he wanted to know how much all of this cost, and when he asked Johnny and found out that his new son-in-law had spent over eight hundred dollars on wholesale food and liquor and that lots more had been donated, he was bedazzled and amazed. He just kept going on and on about how much it cost and how much wine and beer was consumed and how many boxes of cigars were passed out. Obviously, my daddy was not a very sophisticated man. No one ever accused him of having a lot of class.

Daddy handed us a check for five hundred dollars. We knew the check wasn't any good, and that he was doing it for show. Johnny and I knew not to try to cash that check, and we never mentioned it again.

Daddy never commented on how his daughter looked as a young bride. It was hard for my daddy to say complimentary things like that, but he just couldn't stop raving about all the money that everything cost. I didn't care about the money. It didn't matter a whit to me. I loved having a beautiful wedding to celebrate my marriage to Johnny. I was in love with Johnny. That was all that mattered to me.

Long before we were married, Johnny was always coming through for me. When I couldn't quite pay the rent, he offered money to help out. He bought essentials as well as gifts for me. He gave me advice and guidance. When Johnny provided the wedding, I appreciated the wedding, but I didn't really appreciate how special it was for the groom to be doing all of this. It didn't register with me how unusual it was for a teenager to take on such responsibility.

I took what he did for granted. He had always done things for me. Today, when I think back on how this nineteen-year-old kid organized and paid for our wedding, including his bride's wedding gown, and held a reception for hundreds and hundreds of people, I think it is pretty amazing. He was a special man. He still is. I felt so lucky that I was marrying Johnny. After more than forty years, I still feel lucky.

CHAPTER FOUR

Susie Warren Hales

My mama, Susie Warren Hales, was born September 13, 1896, in Evergreen, Alabama. When she was a toddler, her mama died. Susie was raised by her stepmother and grew up with half brothers and sisters. Very little is known about Susie's mother, my grandmother.

Susie was the family beauty. Cherokee ancestry gave her high cheek bones and a regal bearing. Her flawless, olive complexion was a shade richer and deeper than those of her half brothers and sisters. Hazel-green eyes with dark lashes, and heavy, wavy black hair gave her a sophisticated air in impoverished surroundings. She was tiny, barely five feet tall. The stories of her always included, in addition to continued reference to her beauty, comments about how she was the gentle one, the good one, the one others could count on to help out.

Her cousin Lorraine tells that, when Susie's cousin Thelma was in labor with her first child and had nobody to be with her, it was Susie who walked miles in knee-deep snow to help. Folks said she was a "good ol' soul." That's a compliment in the south. I never ever heard a bad thing said about Mama.

Her beauty was recognized by everyone. Village tales tell of a prominent man in their small town taking a shine to her, but he was married, and Susie's daddy put a stop to it. That was when my daddy, Bose Genkins King, entered the picture. He was a sandy-haired, blue-eyed charmer. Everyone called him B.G. He was handsome and full of laughter and fun. He won Mama's hand, and I'm sure, her heart, too.

Mama was the glue that held our family together. She salvaged the fruits and vegetables Daddy brought home from the bruised and rotting produce thrown out by the local grocers. She'd cut away the bad spots and can them so we would have food for winter.

I hungered for stories of my mother's beauty and goodness, about her competence in providing for her family, and about her warmth and love for her children. I was comforted and reassured as I heard these stories again and again. The tired, listless, gray-haired mother I knew radiated none of these traits. The older children remember our mama when she laughed and sang. I do not. In those preteen years when mothers are so important to young girls seeking an example of how to mold their coming womanhood, those stories about my mama helped me fill a void.

My sister Mary tells about the time when she was in the hospital having her tonsils out, and Mama was visiting her. Mama wanted to call Daddy, but she couldn't dial the phone. Finally a nurse came and dialed for her. Mary had to tell her the number. Another time, she told about when Mama had forgotten how to transfer on the bus. Nobody knew it, but Mama was sick even then.

Mama had never been very well. Even before I could remember her, she had been frail. She had tuberculosis when she was a young woman. That was before I was born, but my brothers and sisters told me that we lived in a tent so Mama could have lots of fresh air. Now I realize that if she needed fresh air, we could have opened the windows of a house, and that the family probably lived in a tent because we were so poor.

After she had tuberculosis, she never fully regained her strength. Anna June tells of a time when she and Mama were walking home from church, and Mama just sat down on the curb and said that she couldn't walk any further. She was just too tired to take another step. Anna June was embarrassed and tried to make Mama get up and walk home, but Mama wouldn't move. Finally, Daddy had to come get her. But mostly, Mama was quiet and uncomplaining. She was just there doing things for her family. Everybody took her for granted.

Mama died when she was fifty-two years old, but she looked like a very, very, old woman. Tommy Lou worked in the same hospital where Mama had gone for tests, and she looked up Mama's medical chart. Someone had written, "This woman should never have had children." I always thought it was a pointless statement to make after Mama had delivered nine of us. No wonder she was always tired.

At her funeral, because she had been bedridden for so long, they dressed her in a negligee instead of a dress. A lavender negligee. I will never forget that shimmery, gossamer gown and its elegant color. They had curled my mama's hair. I had never seen her hair curled before, only braided or crudely cut short. Her hair had turned totally white, and now it framed her face in a silver halo of soft waves. They had put makeup on her face, giving vibrant color to her once pallid, expressionless countenance. My mama had never worn makeup, being a Pentecostal and all. After bearing nine children, her body had thickened. Now, in the thinness of her death, her emaciated body looked slender and delicate.

My breath caught short to see her lying there so exquisitely beautiful. My mother looked lovely. Never before in my life had I seen her look lovely. She lay there cushioned by the silken softness of the ivory-cream, satin-lined casket, prettier than any angel from heaven. My own mother. I wanted the world to see her and recognize her beauty. Mixed with the sadness of losing the mother I never had, I felt proud of her elegance and of her beauty. Since the day of her funeral, lavender has been my favorite color.

A few relatives attended the funeral. My sister Mary traveled from faraway Hollywood, but Tommy Lou couldn't make it home. My other sisters, Ruth, Minnie Sue, and Norma Jean, and my brothers, Herschel and Leonard, were there. Frank Hayles,

Mama's half-brother, came from St. Louis. I was impressed that he was there. I'd never met him before, and no one has ever seen or heard of him since. Some of Mama's church friends were there, and various neighbors attended.

After the funeral, we all gathered at the cemetery for the graveside service. I remember the stone Daddy had made for Mama, and I was surprised and concerned that it had his name on it, too, only without the last date for dying, of course. I couldn't stand the thought of my daddy dying, too. Especially now when I felt so alone. He calmed my fears by explaining that it was cheaper to have two names on one stone than to buy two stones. Actually, there was room for three names. For Daddy, saving money and getting a bargain on something was always a big deal. He actually had also bought three cemetery plots, sort of a three-for-one package deal, one for each of them and an extra for whoever died next. Just in case he might have to bury somebody else in the family, he had it covered. The stone and plot were already paid for.

Minnie Sue always said that she was going to be buried in that plot beside her Mama and Daddy. She was, too. Her name is the third name there on the headstone right along with theirs.

At the graveside Daddy pointed to the plot beside Mama's grave and announced with a degree of bravado to show his loyalty to his wife, "Right there, that's where I'm gonna be. I'm gonna be right next to my Susie." And, indeed, that is right where he is today.

Following all the services, everyone came over to the house on Reynolds Street. I remember that there were lots of potted, flowering plants people had brought to us, and we placed them along the edge of the porch and up the steps. I thought they looked so pretty, all those flowers. People brought food, and there was plenty for everyone to eat. Folks were milling around and visiting with one another.

I remember that I wore the yellow plaid suit which had been last year's Easter outfit and, although it was a little small by now, was slated to be worn again for this Easter. I wore it to my mama's funeral instead.

My emotions on that day were complex and confusing to me. While I was sad because my mother died, I was also strangely relieved. An undercurrent of uncomfortable guilt gnawed at me. At the same time, I felt quite grown-up. I was, after all, her youngest child, an important person on an important day.

I think we were all relieved that it was over. We were angry, too. Angry that such a good and kind person, who was so undeserving of all this torture, the bed sores, the stiff body, had to suffer so. People talked of her seizures, and I remembered the times toward the very end of her life when I would be alone with Mama, and she would have a seizure. Her seizures terrified me. I wanted them to stop talking about her seizures, especially here at her funeral.

We could only imagine her pain. No one had any way of knowing how she had really suffered. We only knew that she didn't deserve to go through all that she had gone through.

People chatted about the tragedy of it all and talked angrily about the hospital, about how it happened, and what "they" had done to Mama. Today, I believe deep in my heart that if we had known then what we know now, we would have known that she wasn't going to get well even if nothing had gone wrong at the hospital. She would have just gotten crazy and done strange things and died slowly over the years, bit by bit. Maybe, if we had known, we would not have been so angry .

Everybody ate until they couldn't hold any more food, and then we all posed for pictures there in front of the porch and sitting on the front steps. My daddy, my brothers and sisters, various aunts, uncles, cousins, and some friends, neighbors and I sat or stood in various combinations to have our presence immortalized for the record. Daddy ended up in most of the pictures. He was definitely the star of the afternoon. After all, he was the widower who had cared dutifully for his sick wife through all those difficult years. I am confident Daddy was relieved by her death, but today he was the man who had lost his beloved Susie. And it was Daddy, after all, who had kept the family together. He deserved to be in most of the pictures. He had earned and now basked in the many condolences coming his way. I remember that Mama's funeral was a sadly festive occasion.

I loved my mama, or at least I loved what little I remember of her and all of what I fantasized her to have been. I knew in my heart, buried somewhere in the misty memories of my confused and painful past, that my mama had loved me, too.

My search to find my mother, to know for myself who she truly was, what she was really like, had ended without my ever finding her. The search to find her history had yet to begin.

CHAPTER FIVE

Bose Genkins King

My daddy, Bose Genkins King, was born in Bluefield, West Virginia, on September 24, 1895, the youngest of six children. His smile would melt your heart. He was heart-breaking handsome, with a "devil-may-care" kind of charm. His older sisters had spoiled him rotten, and while he was fun loving, he also was a complainer and cry baby. It was always, "poor me." With Daddy, it was always the other guy's fault, the world owed him a living, and everyone in the world except Bose King had it easy. He envied what others had and was jealous of anyone who had more than he had—except for children, of course.

When Mama was pregnant with their third child, Minnie Sue, Daddy wrote to his sister and said that this was the last kid they were ever going to have. It was clear that Bose King did not want nine children. In that same letter, he said that Susie, my mother, wanted them to send something for the new baby. I can't believe Mama would ever say that. Mama wouldn't ask for anything. Daddy was the one who always thought somebody else should be doing something for him.

I've never been able to figure out just how he managed to think that he wasn't responsible for all those kids he kept having. My daddy believed that people should feel sorry for him for having so many kids and help him out.

I remember him always saying to anyone who would listen, "If you're going to go into business, don't do like I did. I went into the kid business. It's the wrong business to get into." He emphasized the word "wrong" in kind of sing-songy way, and thought he was being clever. His comments made all of us kids feel like we weren't particularly valuable to our daddy.

Daddy refused to carry any insurance, not medical insurance for his family, nor fire insurance for the house, nor car insurance, nor life insurance. He said that he did not believe in giving his money away to someone else and get absolutely nothing back. He felt that was especially true about life insurance. What good would money do him when he was dead? It was a skewed logic, but typical of Bose King.

"I ain't givin' nobody no money an' gettin' nothin' in return. No, siree. They ain't gonna cheat me outta my money," Daddy would rant, as though preaching some great and wise wisdom that only he had seen. Actually, I don't think he ever had any money to be cheated out of.

He resented having the responsibility of a large family, but he did take care of us in his fashion. For as long as I can remember, he worked most of the time. I heard from the older kids that there were often times when Daddy didn't have work, and the family struggled to get by. Daddy wasn't particularly ambitious. He never tried to build his painting business into anything successful. He just took the jobs as they came and did a good job when he went to work. When the boys married, they took jobs for other people and didn't work for themselves. They were excellent painters, but they knew that keeping busy on your own was hard work.

The older kids remember times when there wasn't enough to eat, but I don't. As long as I can remember, we were never hungry. The food wasn't very fancy, but it was food. Often, I remember taking a quarter out of the sugar bowl to go to the corner store to buy milk, bread, and bologna, and that was lunch or dinner, whichever.

Daddy was always good to me. Mama did the spanking, not Daddy. Only once did he hurt me. I was on the front porch one afternoon talking to Johnny's best friend, Joe, and I was supposed to have done some chore in the house. Joe just happened to stop by, so I began talking to him. Daddy asked if I'd finished my chore, and I told him no, but that I'd do it in a minute. He walked over to me, and, right there in front of Joe, he slapped me hard across the face. It stung terribly, but what really hurt me was the humiliation I felt. That's the only time he ever hit me, but I remember it as clearly as if it had happened yesterday. Daddy and the boys fought like wildcats when the boys got older. But Daddy was not the disciplinarian— Mama was.

Daddy loved to have fun, loved holidays, loved picnics. He would hoard fireworks until the 4th of July arrived and then have a big display for all of us. I suspect now, it was mostly because he loved fireworks. He made things for us, slides and a merry-go-round in the yard. He would walk on his hands and play like a kid. I remember when he used to take us swimming.

He didn't get too involved with being a parent. We were left pretty much on our own, except for being expected to do the chores he told us to do. Other than that, he never knew or seemed to care what we were doing. We went pretty much wherever we wanted to go. We went to bed when we wanted to and ate whenever we were hungry. There was nobody who cared if we did our school work or not, or even if we went to school. It didn't matter to anybody when we came and went.

Daddy stuck by us and didn't run off and leave us when Mama was sick, and he helped take care of her. You can believe that he didn't want to! I gave him lots of credit for hanging in there like he did. I don't know why I was so impressed because Daddy didn't leave us, as though it was perfectly reasonable for a man to abandon his family if everything wasn't going to suit him. I know now that a father is supposed to take care of his family, but then, I thought he did this heroic thing, sort of like I really didn't deserve having a daddy stay and take care of me when he didn't really want to. I always realized that he resented being stuck raising a bunch of kids he didn't want. Somehow, I felt responsible for his plight. Yet, in spite of all his faults and shortcomings, I loved my daddy and carry a warm spot in my heart for him to this day.

Daddy died in 1959 of cancer. He was sixty-four years old. I remember the day of Mama's funeral in vivid detail. I can't even recall if Daddy had a funeral or not.

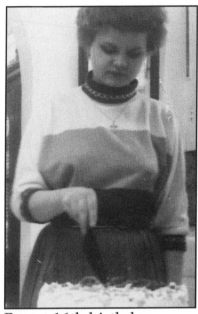
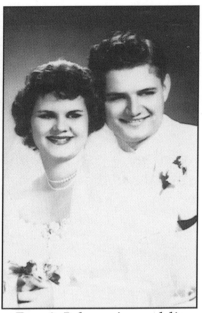

Bea at 16th birthday   Bea & Johnny's wedding

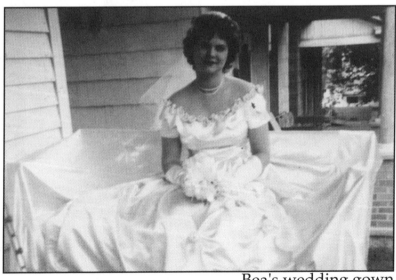

Bea's wedding gown

CHAPTER SIX

Herschel

Herschel was the first one of my brothers and sisters to succumb to Alzheimer's disease, although at the time, it didn't occur to any of us to make a connection between Herschel's early forgetfulness and Mama's illness. When Herschel became ill, we still didn't think of Mama as having had a disease that somebody else might have. Also, Herschel's behavior was different. Most of us remembered Mama as being almost in a coma, the way she was for the final years of her life. What was happening in Herschel's life was completely misunderstood, and he was judged as having some kind of flaw in his character. People felt Herschel should be able to control his actions, and he just wouldn't.

When I was growing up, Herschel was more like another adult in the house rather than a brother. He was seventeen when I was born and had long since stopped going to school. Instead, he went to work just like Daddy did. He lived at home until the war broke out. He was one of the first ones drafted and spent the next five years in the army. I didn't miss him. Our house was so full of people, it was difficult to miss anybody.

Herschel was the epitome of the "tall-dark-and-handsome" matinee idol of his day. He was a quiet and gentle man, but he could also be quite playful. He and Daddy were forever cooking up some kind of practical joke or pranks to play on someone. Although he was very handsome, Herschel was painfully shy and never had a steady girl friend until he met Midge, the woman he would marry. Hidden behind his shyness was a deep insecurity. It bothered him that he had never studied in school and didn't have an education.

Three times during his life, Herschel had almost died. When he was in his early teens, he almost drowned. A few years later, he was accidentally shot in the face and carried the scar all his life. The war changed Herschel. In the army, he was buried alive, but survived. He was the only one in his battalion who survived the war, and he always seemed to feel guilty to have lived when his buddies had not. In his day-to-day life, he suppressed his inner turmoil. Herschel rarely mentioned those experiences, yet their memory haunted him, and rarely, very rarely, he turned to alcohol in an attempt to obliterate the pain. His bouts of drunkenness brought out a wild, violent, angry man.

I remember him destroying the kitchen during one drunken rage, tearing the cabinets off the walls and throwing them hard against the floor. He terrified me when he drank. But most of the time, he was just

Herschel, easygoing on the surface, conscientious about his work, and gentle with me, his little sister.

When he was discharged from the army, he bought one of the first television sets on the market, a black-and-white model with a seven-inch screen. I remember the pictures were often snowy, but we watched nonetheless in total fascination. Having a television made us kind of like celebrities in our neighborhood, and I felt quite privileged. No one else had a television. "Howdy Doody" was a favorite program. Johnny used to tease me that he came over to my house just to watch our TV and not to see me. I knew better.

Herschel also bought a convertible. Televisions and convertibles were definitely rich folks' toys. I thought my oldest brother was very worldly. On rare occasions, he let me ride with him with the top down, and the wind would blow against my face and whip my hair around.

When Herschel was thirty-two years old, he moved to California and married Midge, a woman several years older. Midge had an eighteen-year-old daughter, and he and Midge had a son whom Herschel adored. They named their son Herschel after his father and called him Shelly.

Herschel settled in, a married man with a family and a steady job. He bought his first house on the veteran's home loan program with a dollar down. Herschel loved that house and worked on it all the time. He was a skillful painter whom people could rely on to do a good job. Like Daddy, he also hung wallpaper and did miscellaneous carpentry jobs. Herschel was known as a kind, decent, hard working man who took pride in doing things well. He could be counted on. Other than on those rare, nightmarish binges, Herschel never drank. Most of the time, he was a dedicated family man, gentle and devoted to his wife and child. His life was going well. At least that's what I have been told. I did not see him for years at a time, so I don't know first hand.

Years later Midge told us about how Herschel had changed. He began to forget things, to become disoriented and not know where he was, to forget to show up for jobs, to arrive at a job site and find he had forgotten his tools, or he would forget what he was supposed to do when he got there. He would wander around bewildered, and finally go home. Herschel was the foreman of his painting crew. Each day the boss would give him a work order of things to be done the next day. Herschel would bring home the work order, and Midge would read it and explain where he was supposed to be and what he was supposed to do. Herschel got to where he could no longer remember what Midge had told him. It became difficult to hold a job. Lack of work created financial problems, which added to the family's stress and tension.

The changes in his behavior came about gradually. Poorly done work. Confusion about what had to be done. Insidious changes. Was he going through some sort of mid-life crisis? After all, we all forget things. But it was more than forgetting. His personality was changing. His moods were extreme. Herschel became more and more difficult.

As things became worse, Midge told of Herschel's headaches and his confusion. From time to time, he would lash out at his family, accusing them of doing crazy things they had not done. My mama had died before Midge and Herschel were married, and Herschel didn't talk much about Mama. Midge didn't really know any details about Mama's illness, and she never thought for a minute that Herschel might have what his mama had.

She only knew that the changes in her husband's behavior taxed her patience. Herschel was in his forties and looked normal, but his behavior was strange. He would get lost walking in the neighborhood and be frightened when Midge or his son Shelly would find him. He kept asking to go home to Kansas City. He hadn't lived there for almost twenty years. Midge shared with us how Herschel would talk about the war, often rambling on in a disconnected babble, and how he would cry and cry. His endless sobbing worried her. She felt helpless and at a loss about what to do for him.

It was sometime in 1970, when Midge was at her wit's end, that I suggested Herschel come visit us for a week so she could have a break. Today, we call that "respite care." Other than feeding my mother, I had never been a caregiver, and Mama was a vegetable, not a trouble maker. I had no idea of what to expect. I also had no idea of what I was getting myself into.

Having Herschel with us was an eye opener and my first lesson in appreciating the tremendous burden carried by caregivers. I was managing some condominiums at the time. My brother looked physically normal, healthy and handsome, strong and fit, so I decided to ask him to help me do some of the cleaning to ready an empty unit for rental.

"Herschel, could I get you to come with me tomorrow and help me clean a condo? I could sure use you," I said to him. He mumbled something in response, which I assumed meant that he was willing to help. I really looked forward to having a strong man do some of the heavy work.

We talked in the car as I drove. Actually, I talked, and Herschel sort of mumbled or grunted. When we arrived, he carried the vacuum inside for me, sat it on the carpet, and stood there with a blank look on his face.

"If you could start vacuuming in the bedroom, that would be great. I'll start cleaning here in the kitchen." I spoke to him cheerfully, thinking that this cleanup job would be short work with two people. I was in for one big surprise.

Herschel continued to stand there and then began to fiddle with the cord, undoing it from the handle and then trying to put it back. I watched him and my heart sank. It was obvious that he was trying, but had no idea how to use the vacuum. I tried unsuccessfully to show him. He was making no connection between what I was explaining and what he was expected to do, so I decided to give him another simple job. It was soon clear that doing any kind of work was beyond him. It came as a shock to me when I began to realize just how bad things had become for my sister-in-law.

The week he stayed with us was a nightmare. Herschel would wander around our house, confused with the unfamiliarity of the place. He would disappear, and I would find him in the garage, rummaging through the tool drawers and boxes of things we had stored there. He left things strewn about as he removed them. He would walk into the kid's room and stare at them, as though trying to figure out who they were. My kids had seldom seen their uncle and were scared to death of him and his weird behavior.

"What's the matter with Uncle Herschel, Mom? Why is he doing this anyway?" young John asked. Kim and Wendy steered clear of him whenever possible. I tried to explain, but didn't do a very good job of it. For one thing, I didn't really want to deal with what was happening. I certainly didn't want to plant the idea with the children that their mother might someday be doing the same weird things. Neither did I want to entertain the idea myself.

Herschel would wander through the house, obviously wanting something. He couldn't explain what he wanted, and I couldn't figure it out. I was running water in the sink one day, and he wanted a drink, but he couldn't tell me. He came over to the sink and tried to drink the water out of the faucet. I gave him a glass.

He'd watch himself in the mirror and talk to the person he called his friend. When we left to go somewhere, Herschel would ask if he could bring his friend.

"What friend?" I asked him.

"Here," he responded and took me to the mirror. "Him. He's my friend. That's him right there," he said, pointing to his reflection. It was funny and sad and scary all at the same time.

Herschel kept repeating, "When's she comin' after me? When's she gonna come get me?" Once, I couldn't help myself, and I asked, "Who, Herschel? Who's comin'?" And he said, "Her." He couldn't remember his wife's name. I broke down and wept.

That evening in the shower, he cried out in panic. Johnny rushed in to see what the problem was and found that Herschel had tried to put his shorts on over his head and his legs through the sleeves of his T-shirt and was stuck. Thank, God, Johnny was home. I don't know what I would have done if I'd had to wrestle with my naked, wet brother, trying to disentangle him from the trap he had made for himself.

The entire week was like this. Herschel went into our next-door neighbor's house, just walked right in and poured himself a cup of cold coffee in a dirty cup that was left on the sink. To complicate matters, this happened around midnight. The wife was scared to death when she saw him and screamed loudly enough to wake the dead. Herschel, probably more frightened than she was, scurried right out of her kitchen, coffee cup and all, and came back to our house. She called the police. It was a mess, trying to explain to my neighbor and to the police. I'd never had such a horrible week in my entire life.

At the end of the week, Midge came and picked him up. I felt guilty that I was so glad to see her, knowing she would have to take him home and deal with him everyday. I wondered how she did it. How on earth was she surviving this chaos? My heart went out to her. I told her about Herschel's friend in the mirror.

"Oh, yeah," she replied, "he does it all the time. He calls me to come in the bathroom, and he points to the mirror so I can meet his friend. Whenever we go somewhere, he asks me if his friend can come. I tell him sure and give him a pocket mirror to take with us. I gotta confess, Bea, I like that little ol' mirror buddy 'cause he keeps Herschel busy and happy for hours. And heaven knows, he isn't hurtin' nothin'. If he isn't hurtin' nothin', believe me, I jus' let it be."

For a long time, Herschel had complained of headaches, and Midge took him back to the VA hospital. He was examined by two doctors, and both felt that the problem was high blood pressure. They gave him medication, but the problems continued.

One day he fainted at work, and they called Midge to come get him and take him home. Once home, Herschel turned to his wife and said, "Somethin's wrong with me." Midge said that he looked so confused and troubled. Her heart ached for him. He was fifty-one years old, a man in the prime of his life, and his mind was crumbling within while his world was crumbling around him.

Midge took him back to the VA hospital where she felt there were competent doctors, and Herschel would get good care. This time the examination took most of the day. They could find nothing wrong with him physically, but the doctors suggested he see a neurologist. The appointment was for one o'clock the next afternoon.

Midge and Herschel arrived early and ate lunch before going to the hospital. Once they were in the examination room, the doctor began asking Herschel questions.

"Who is President of the United States, Herschel?" he asked. Herschel looked confused. He did not know.

"Can you tell me when you were born? When's your birthday?"

Again, Herschel looked blankly at the doctor and said nothing.

"How old are you, Herschel?" Again, no response. Midge told the doctor that her husband was fifty-one.

"Is your father living?" asked the doctor. Herschel looked at his interrogator, a confused expression on his face. Then he looked at his wife. Midge answered the question.

"What did he die of?" The doctor continued. Again, Herschel did not know. Midge answered.

"And your mother? Is she living, Herschel?" Another confused, blank stare from Herschel. Another response from Midge.

"His mama died before I met an' married Herschel, so I never knew her," she told the doctor. "I think she had some sorta problem, but I don't really know much about it. Herschel doesn't talk about her at all."

The doctor changed the subject. "What did you have for lunch, Herschel?" he asked.

"I never ate," Herschel responded. Midge was now very discouraged. She told the doctor that they had already eaten lunch.

"A cheeseburger and fries," she explained.

The doctor wanted Herschel admitted to the hospital as soon as possible and asked Midge for Herschel's mother's name and her doctor so that he could send for her medical records. She contacted our sister Ruth and got the name of Susie King's doctor.

Herschel went into the hospital on the following day. They continued to administer psychological tests, none of which Herschel remembered taking. When they had trouble keeping him in bed, they tried restraining him. Finally, he was placed in a strait jacket, but on several occasions, he was able to work himself free.

His teeth were very bad, and Midge asked the doctors about doing some dental work for him while he was in the hospital. Shortly after he had been admitted, Midge visited him and found him covered with blood and there was blood all over the bedding. She called hysterically for the nurses. It turned out that they had pulled his teeth and were fitting him for dentures, and he had begun to bleed again. Midge was relieved. Considering the condition of his teeth, she was grateful to have them taken care of.

Doctors at the VA hospital diagnosed Herschel as having Alzheimer's disease and recommended that Midge take him to Fort Miley in San Francisco where they did a biopsy of Herschel's brain tissue. This procedure is rarely done today, since it is very painful. After the biopsy surgery, the doctors told Midge that Herschel would never work again and that she should explore some means of supporting herself and the family. They suggested that she look into Social Security or veteran's benefits. They did not explain what options she might have in providing care for her husband.

Midge was in a state of shock. It had not occurred to her that Herschel was now incapable of working. She must now accept the fact that her husband would never recover. After the surgery Herschel's decline was the worst and most rapid it had been during the entire duration of the disease.

He was released from the hospital, and Midge took him home. One night, shortly after he came home, Midge was awakened by Herschel standing over her quivering with rage and shaking his fist close to his wife's face.

"I'm going to knock the hell out of you!" Herschel shouted angrily, his voice was seething with anger. His eyes had a crazed expression. Herschel had never spoken to Midge that way before, and she lay frozen with fear. Not too long after that incident, Herschel went into his son Shelly's room and, as Shelly lay on the bed, Herschel jumped on him and began flailing his fists in the air and swearing at him. Both attacks were totally out of character. Shelly was the apple of Herschel's eye. He lived for Shelly. This stranger was not the devoted husband and father they knew.

Frightened and unable to care for her husband and having neither the knowledge nor skills with which to cope, Midge made the most difficult decision of her life. She knew she had no way of handling the vast problems created by Herschel. She also knew that she and her son could well be in danger. She placed her husband in the Napa State Mental Hospital in Napa, California, not far from their home in Vallejo. They had been married for twenty-one years.

Almost two decades later, when support groups and respite care were commonplace, Midge expressed regret that none had been available to her or Shelly when they had needed them. Looking back, she would have preferred to care for her husband at home had she known more about the disease and about what to do for and expect from her difficult husband. If only there had been someone for her to talk to, someone who could have told her what the future held, someone to ease her guilt, or to help carry the load, maybe she could have cared for him at home. But at that time, there had been no place for her to turn.

Midge visited Herschel regularly and always brought him a malted milk drink and his favorite Snickers candy bar, and he would smile when he saw them. Midge was never sure whether he knew she was his wife or not. She comforted herself that at least he knew she was someone who loved and cared for him. Still, it hurt that it seemed Herschel was far more interested in the malt drink and candy bar than he was in the person bringing the gifts.

It is ironic that on three occasions, Herschel narrowly survived death only to live long enough to succumb to the tortuous death from Alzheimer's disease. He died on March 28, 1972. He was fifty-four.

At Herschel's funeral, his younger brother Leonard, recently divorced and with his new girlfriend, sat apart from the family. In spite of their difference in age, Herschel and Leonard had been very close. When people spoke of the good times the brothers had shared, Leonard could remember none of them. I suspected then that Leonard might be following in his brother's footsteps.

CHAPTER SEVEN

Jack

Kimberly and Wendy were teenagers and young John was in the first grade at school, so the constant caring for kids had eased considerably. I was working outside the home at various jobs, but in spite of this, the late 1960s were difficult years for me. I felt isolated and alone. An unsettling, haunting emptiness pervaded me and refused to leave. I was in my mid-thirties. I was constantly wondering if there had been symptoms of the early stages of Alzheimer's that we hadn't recognized in Herschel and Minnie Sue when they were in their mid-thirties?

I examined my every flaw. Where did I put the car keys? Why did I forget to put bread on the list of things for Johnny to bring home from the market? Was young John's dental appointment at 2:00 or 2:30? Why didn't I write it down? Was this the day I was supposed to pick up Wendy after school? My purse, where on earth did I put my purse?

I lost my temper easily with my kids and with Johnny. I knew it was because this was the beginning of the end. My depression deepened.

Although I genuinely enjoyed some of the jobs I held, none filled the void that ate away at my middle. Johnny was working longer hours than ever, and I felt abandoned by him and felt that I needed more of his attention. I was evidently getting more of his attention than I gave him credit for, because in 1970, I found that I was pregnant. Instead of feeling joy at the prospect of another baby, I fell further into my bleak and heavy depression. How could I ever take care of another child when I was sure I was beginning to lose my mind and shortly, would lose it altogether? Young John had grown into a cheerful, independent little boy. He would be seven by the time this baby was born. I dreaded the thought of the demanding care needed by an infant. Having a toddler again who couldn't dress himself, who wasn't toilet trained, who had no little brothers and sisters to play with and hence, would need much more of my time, overwhelmed me.

But most of all, I was haunted by the thought of not being able to take proper care of another child. Would this baby go through what I had gone through? It would probably be much worse than what I had experienced. My behavior would probably be more like Herschel's. And like Minnie Sue's. We were hearing more and more about the strange things Minnie Sue was doing. She couldn't hold a job. She would lash out at people. She couldn't talk clearly. She swore. Minnie

Sue had never used bad language. She definitely was not herself.

If I began to act like either of them, how could I possibly take care of this baby? How could I even take care of the children I already had? I would be thirty-six when the baby came, just three years younger than my mother had been when I was born. By the time the child was four or five, my mind could very well be completely gone. How could I put my other children in a situation of having to take on the work and responsibility of raising a little brother or sister? I saw no other way out. I would have an abortion.

Johnny supported me. He didn't encourage me. He just supported me. He knew the terror I was feeling. I talked with friends at church. They sympathized and agreed that, with the history of family illness and my certainty that I was going to be next in line, I was taking a wise, practical, and responsible step. One of these friends had worked for the health department and suggested that I go to Sacramento to the state health department for counseling. I decided to go. I would stay with Minnie Sue's daughter, Anna Sue, who lived in Sacramento. Johnny drove me down. My heart was heavy.

Waiting in the stark halls of the state buildings, I kept pondering my decision. In my head, I knew it was the right thing to do. In my heart, I wasn't so sure. The wait was long. I hadn't been to a public health office before and didn't know that the wait for public services is always long. I shifted in my seat and read through still another worn magazine missing crucial pages of articles that didn't hold my interest anyway. I watched the people waiting, some sitting, others standing. I watched them come and go, and wondered if I dared give up my chair to walk up and down the hall and stretch the kinks out of my back. The thought of not having a seat to return to and spending the next hour or two standing quickly erased the temptation of taking a short stroll. I continued to sit. And sit.

At last my turn came. I was ushered in to see the obstetrician. After being set up on that wonderful table that all women have experienced and hate, the doctor left. I waited, Finally, he returned and examined me. I knew I was pregnant. The doctor in Tahoe had told me.

"You're definitely pregnant," he said, and then added, "Who is the father?"

"My husband!" I responded sharply. I was angry and humiliated. Johnny was the father. Just who did he think he was to be asking me such a question? He was oblivious to my indignation. He finished his examination. Everything was normal. I got down off my perch and told my story. He concurred with my decision, although he didn't seem to care one way or the other. He explained all the gruesome details of the procedure, how it would be suction and all that. I shuddered.

My next appointment was with the psychiatrist. Again, I waited, still seething over the obstetrician's comment. My name was finally called. The doctor was a small man wearing thick glasses and scarcely looked at me. He listened and scribbled notes and nodded. He also agreed that my decision was sound and explained that there was a three-day waiting period after which I would be scheduled to return and have the procedure done. It all appeared routine. Here I was, making the most difficult decision of my life, and nobody seemed to care at all. Exhausted, I returned to my niece's apartment.

There something happened to change my decision. Anna Sue is my sister Minnie Sue's daughter. She was twenty-six then and pregnant with her first child. Like so many new mothers, she was thrilled at the prospect of having a baby. We were sure that her mother Minnie Sue was suffering with Alzheimer's disease, yet Anna Sue had no fear whatsoever. I felt cowardly and ashamed.

Her apartment was filled with baby things. A secondhand crib had been repainted and filled with baby blankets and stuffed toys. A bassinet was adorned with yellow ribbons to be ready for either a boy or a girl. The changing table had diapers and baby clothes stacked neatly on the shelf below, while the top held baby oil, powder, cloths and Q tips. I couldn't stand seeing all the baby things. Anna Sue was ready and eager. She was excited. And although she said very little to me, it was quite clear that she did not think very highly of my decision not to carry my baby to term.

Surrounded by her exuberance about her new baby and what I saw as her courage to have a child with no thought given to either herself or the baby becoming a victim of the disease made me ashamed. Suddenly I could not go through with having an abortion. There were two more days until the scheduled appointment, but I had to get out of there immediately. I placed a desperate call to Johnny and, talking through tears, told him to come get me now. He couldn't get enough time off immediately, and I refused to wait for another day when he could come, so Anna Sue drove me half way to my home in Tahoe, and Johnny drove the other half to meet me. I talked nonstop on the trip home, telling Johnny again and again about my decision, and why I had changed my mind. Bless him always. He as usual, supported me. What was right with me was right with him. After all, I was the one who was pregnant.

Often, I have thanked God for that waiting period. On March 16, 1971, I gave birth to a baby boy, Jack Wayne Gorman. He was perfect. He was beautiful. Love for this infant washed over me in torrents. I felt such joy to hold him, and I shuddered to think that I had come so close to not giving birth to this precious child. His birth was special in another way. When I had my older three children, I had been under anesthetic and slept through each delivery, unconscious of their arrivals. I had a spinal with Jack and was awake when he was born. I will never forget the thrill of holding my new son when he first arrived.

I have thanked God for this baby and believe that I would never have forgiven myself had I gone through with the abortion. Jack and I have always been especially close. Recently, I talked with him about how I was devastated by my pregnancy with him, and of the decision I made, and how I changed my mind. We both cried. He understood. I had always felt guilty that I had never told him. Now was the time for me to share what I had gone through. I didn't want him reading about it in the book. It was an emotional time for us, but it brought renewed closeness, too. We were both pleased with the outcome. Both of us are glad that I changed my mind!

CHAPTER EIGHT

Out of the Darkness

Shortly after Johnny and I were married, we moved to Aurora, Colorado, a suburb of Denver. There Johnny and his father were partners in a grocery store and later, they also opened a meat market. I had always wanted to move to California where my sisters and brothers lived. Tommy Lou wrote glowing letters about sunshine and palm trees and red tile roofs and Spanish stucco. She raved about the warm weather, especially in winter. I pictured California as being only slightly less wonderful than heaven, but Johnny didn't like California. It was too crowded for him. Too impersonal. Johnny likes small, friendly towns where people know each other and speak to each other when they pass on the sidewalk.

We lived in the suburbs of Denver for almost thirteen years. Johnny eventually bought out his father, and we owned the meat market, small grocery store called Gorman's Superette, a motel, and several other businesses. We were both active in the community. Our girls took tap and ballet. John Jr. was too young to be involved in sports. I was active in the PTA, and Johnny was a member of the Jaycees and Chamber of Commerce. Johnny was chosen "Business Man of the Week." He ran the businesses, and I ran errands for him and kept the household going.

Winters were harsh. Summers were short. Denver was not my favorite place. We suffered a series of setbacks in business, but the final blows came when we were burglarized three times, on Thanksgiving, Christmas, and again on New Year's Eve. These are the most profitable days of the year for our types of businesses. Our insurance did not pay, due to a technicality. The young men who committed the crime were found guilty and sent to jail. We didn't retrieve a dime and were never able to fully recover. After years of hard work, we were struggling again. Nothing seemed to be going right in Colorado. Johnny and I decided to make a fresh start somewhere else. Since I had always wanted to live in California, now was my chance.

On a previous trip, we had gone through Lake Tahoe during the summer, and Johnny thought it was the most beautiful place he had ever seen. Johnny would agree to settle in Tahoe. It wasn't my favorite spot, but I thought it would be an improvement over the cold winters in Denver, so in 1968, we headed west. Little did I know that I was trading one set of freezing winters for another.

We took a financial beating when we sold our lovely, three-thousand-square-foot, five bedroom, brick home and moved into what at best could be called a cottage. There was a cluster of motel-like cottages located in Lolly's Lodge. I will never forget Lolly's Lodge. Johnny and I, our three kids and our dog Peaches moved into one of them. Kim was twelve, Wendy was nine, and John Jr. was five. Peaches had evidently been busy giving a loving good-bye to a male friend of hers in Colorado, and, unbeknownst to us, was pregnant when we arrived in our new quarters. Before long, she surprised us by adding six adorable, un-housebroken puppies to our already crowded household.

Our new home had two small bedrooms and a large, walk-in closet. The closet served as Kim's bedroom. The other two kids took one bedroom, and Johnny and I took the other. We were more than cozy, but our spirits were high. We were making a new start in a new place.

Soon we moved to a larger place and, with the exception of one trip back to Denver where Jack was born, we settled into the Tahoe community. Johnny got a job with a major supermarket chain and moved rapidly up through the ranks. I stayed home with the kids.

Lake Tahoe is a place of awe inspiring beauty with fragrant pines and colorful manzanita. Lush ferns cluster in rock crevices bordering clear, rushing mountain streams. Mammoth granite rock outcroppings accent towering mountains as they rise like royalty clothed in icy ermine ruling their kingdom below. This picturesque town of log buildings nestles at the lake's edge. From azure blue to emerald green, the pure, clear waters of Lake Tahoe, gleaming in gem-like splendor, lie cradled in the arms of the forest in picture-post-card perfection.

I hated it. I hated living there with a passion. We had visited Tahoe in the summer. It was sunny and warm and bustling with happy activity. We moved there in the fall. It was a ghost town by comparison. The winter snows arrived and blanketed the town for up to eight, long months. Winters in Denver were mild by comparison.

By winter, skiers flocked to the resorts, but I didn't ski. I struggled to put chains on the tires of the car so that I, a mediocre driver at best, could drive the kids to school or to the doctor or the dentist over slick, icy, treacherous, mountain roads. I bundled up little Jack in boots and hats and coats and mittens and scarves for outside play and unbundled him again for frequent potty breaks. I had a house full of restless kids who were tired of playing in the cold outdoors and too full of energy to settle down inside the house. I had a house full of kids who argued and bickered and teased each other mercilessly.

Dreary months without sunshine depressed me. Although my kids were normal, healthy kids, their constant haranguing depressed me. After years of twisted behavior and suffering, my brother Herschel was now dead from the effects of Alzheimer's disease. Minnie Sue was in the final stages. Although none of us realized it at the time, Leonard was in the early stages of the disease. Even if we had noticed it, none of us would have wanted to admit it. If I had admitted that Leonard was getting "Mama's disease," I would have been more certain and more afraid than ever that I was getting it too. As it was, I was frightened enough that I would be next. Every time I was distraught or harried, as any mother with a bunch of lively kids often is, I knew the disease was beginning to invade my mind.

Johnny was gone all the time. He was a good provider, but he was also a workaholic. His employer thought that was fine, but it left me with most of the responsibility for the day-to-day care of the kids. Winter brought bouts of depression. I felt empty, and I could not understand why. I had four bright, healthy children and a supportive, loving husband. I couldn't understand what was wrong with me.

Many times I morbidly fantasized running my car off a cliff and ending my suffering once and for all. I wanted to die and be done with it. At times the thought of dying obsessed me. Goodness knows, located high in the Sierra Mountains, the Lake Tahoe area offered plenty of cliffs for me to choose from if I wanted to end it all. I could erase my problems and myself in dizzying crash. It was a convenient and comforting fantasy.

One desolate afternoon, young John and Wendy were feuding. Baby Jack was now three, and he was fussing and crying with all the confusion. I had reached the end of my rope. Kim, who by this time was in college, had come home for the Christmas break, and instead of staying at home with the family where she belonged, she was staying with her boyfriend. I didn't approve. That sounds too mild. I disapproved big time. I felt that I had failed as a parent to teach her the right values. Failed because she would no longer listen to me. The whole episode made me extremely distraught, but when kids are in college, they don't do what you want them to do. They do what they want to do. There's not much you can tell college kids. My life, my kids, everything was out of control.

I remember sitting on the couch, terribly depressed, staring at the hypnotic dance of endlessly falling snow. It fell in a silent, swirling onslaught, amassing mounds of deadly white, icy fluff in which to bury me. Herschel's bizarre actions plagued me. Minnie Sue's mind was now completely gone. I was coming up on forty, the dreaded decade when members of my family began this craziness, and I was constantly haunted by wondering when this curse would begin with me or, worse yet, if maybe it had already begun.

Something snapped. I got up, walked out of the house, got into the car, and started to drive. Wendy was a teenager, so she could look after the baby. I had to get away. I was like the kid that says, "I'm gonna run away from home," or, "I'm gonna kill myself, and then you'll be sorry." I felt sorry for myself, and I just couldn't take it any more. I left the house, determined to drive the car off a cliff. Instead of finding my way to a cliff, nearby and handy, I drove around aimlessly and, seemingly without thinking, pulled the car into our church parking lot. I turned off the engine, sat there in the car, and shivered.

The Catholic church in Tahoe is a small, log structure. I was freezing cold and thought I'd better go inside where it was warmer. I walked to the church door and was surprised to find it open. Entering, I sat down. Candles were burning, but the church was empty. There was not a sound. I didn't kneel, didn't cross myself, didn't pray. I just sat down. My body was numb from the cold and from my emotional drain. The warmth I was looking for eluded me. Inside the church was almost as cold as it had been in the unheated car. I sat there, frozen to the bone and still as death. I listened and studied the Cross and Jesus. That was all I looked at. I was aware of the flickering candles, but my eyes were transfixed on the Cross and on Jesus. I was listening for somebody to give me direction. I didn't actually ask for direction. I just listened for what seemed to me an interminably long time. Just how long, I didn't know or don't remember. It was brutally cold, and I remember that I was finally so chilled that I couldn't sit there any longer. I walked out of the church into the dismal, overcast late afternoon. It was snowing. It was always snowing. I felt trapped by all that snow. I wanted to scream.

Getting into the car, and without making a conscious decision, I drove directly to the public library. It was as though I were being given direction, not from a voice, but in my mind's eye or my mind's ear. Once inside the library, without asking anyone for anything, I walked directly to the religious section. I did not browse through the books. I just picked one off the shelf, stared at the picture on the book jacket, and then checked it out. That book changed my life.

That book was *The Power of Positive Thinking* by Dr. Norman Vincent Peale. I couldn't put it down. It was as though it became an extension of my arm. Throughout the book were quotes from the Bible. The book kept referring to scripture. Catholics didn't read the Bible much in those days. Now they read the Bible more, but then, reading the Bible was new to me. I began looking up and reading scriptures.

Dr. Peale's book listed other books, and I read them. They fed a hunger in me. They quenched a thirst. I couldn't get enough. While reading, I started to think differently. As my thoughts changed, I changed, and my life changed. I became stronger. Much, much stronger.

I know now that the Lord listened to me in my desperation, and on that snowy afternoon in a small, frigid, log church in Lake Tahoe, the Lord reached out to me and guided me. I didn't know it then, but I know it now.

Nothing on the outside had changed. From all outward appearances, my life was the same. Herschel was dead. Minnie Sue was failing rapidly. Leonard was taking his first steps along the tortuous path leading him to his death. I still could well be next. Johnny was still a workaholic. I still had four wonderful, but trying kids, and I still carried most of the responsibility for their care, but I was different. I had made a deep and personal connection with my God, and with Jesus, and I was no longer alone. For the first time in a very long time, I experienced joy in my life. Pure, exhilarating, exquisite joy!

I was also rapidly becoming bored with the Catholic Church. I needed to find more. I needed something that touched me personally. It was my son John who opened the door for me. He was very active in the church, serving as an altar boy and attending the youth programs. John asked me one day if I knew they had a prayer group at St. Teresa. I didn't.

"I've never seen anything about a prayer group in the church bulletin," I said. "Do they keep it a secret?"

"No, but they don't print it in the bulletin. I don't think it's a very big group, but I'm sure it would be something you'd like," he assured me.

He was right. If I hadn't found that group, I feel sure that I would have left my church, but I did find that wonderful prayer group, and I didn't leave. I joined them, and we met once a week in the chapel.

The prayer group was praying for me to receive the gifts of the spirit. I remember in the beginning that they wanted me to speak in tongues, which is one gift of the spirit, but I didn't want to. It made me very uncomfortable, I think it was because my mother spoke in tongues in her Pentecostal church, and it was scary to me when I was a little girl. I couldn't bring myself to speak in tongues.

The women in the prayer group kept praying for me, but nothing much happened. I became convinced that I was a lost cause and started to wonder why they even bothered to continue. I began to wonder if maybe I shouldn't be there, that maybe I didn't belong in this group after all. I considered not coming anymore.

Midst my doubt, a new woman joined. She had been what was called a "traditional" Catholic and had never even heard of things like speaking in tongues. The group was praying for me when she was the one who was resting in the spirit. She slumped to the floor, helpful arms easing her down. She was lying on the floor, saying over and over,

"This is wonderful! This is wonderful! Oh, oh. This is wonderful."

She was in ecstasy. It looked as though she got zapped instead of me. When it was over, she said that it was the most beautiful and peaceful thing that had ever happened to her. She went on and on describing the wonder of her experience. She asked the group what had happened to her and was told that she was resting in the Spirit. Although the group had been praying for me, the Spirit had gone to her.

I believe I needed to see that. I had never seen anything like it before. It was a powerful meeting. After that, it didn't make any difference to me or to anyone else if I didn't want to speak in tongues. If I wanted to, that was fine. If I didn't, that was fine, too. It didn't have to be one way or the other. Together we studied the Bible, and my commitment to God deepened.

Nobody came to my door and asked me if I wanted to be saved. A person can find God without anyone else being involved. I had begun my journey to God on that afternoon when, desperate and alone, I had started out to drive off a cliff and instead, I ended up sitting in church. It was a very personal thing. When all of this was happening, I didn't realize what was going on. It wasn't until later that I could look back and understand with absolute clarity that God was guiding me.

Although my initial step was taken alone, I have found it helpful and joyful to be with others who shared the same experience. Joining this prayer group was vital to me. It strengthened the foundation for my trust in God, for my renewed, unshakeable faith, and in the joy I felt in knowing Jesus in a deeply personal way.

As I continued to read God's word, I grew unmistakably stronger in every way, not just spiritually, but emotionally, and even physically. The overwhelming challenges I faced no longer devastated me. Fear of my future gave way to a determination to do something with my life. My life had purpose. Hopelessness was transformed into hope. My family welcomed the change in me, and I wanted to announce my newfound joy to the entire world. I wanted to shout it out from the roof tops.

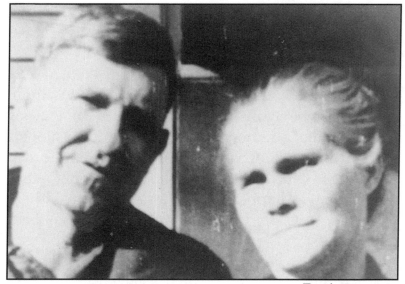

Bea's parents

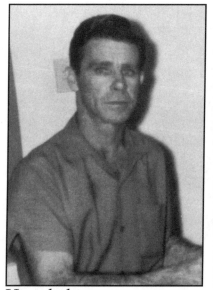

Herschel

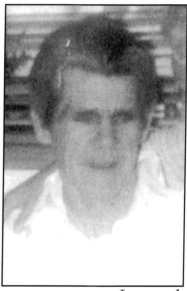

Leonard

CHAPTER NINE

Beginning the Search

With researchers finally acknowledging a definite possibility of a familial link in at least some Alzheimer's cases, I knew I must find out all I could about my mother's family history. I began by asking questions, and from there, I wrote to genealogy organizations, to county records departments, to libraries, to wherever I could think of and asked for microfilm to be sent to Reno. I would then make a trip to Reno and spend days looking over these records trying to find out about Mama's family. Johnny and I trekked from southern town to southern town looking into old records of births and deaths.

When someone told us we might find something in Evergreen, Alabama, off we went to Evergreen. Another lead resulted in another trip. I learned to call or write ahead of time and ask for the microfilm to be available. Then I would go to the town and spend hour after long hour for days on end, trying to find when and how my grandmother had died. We followed every lead, no matter how sketchy. I was driven to learn about Mama's parents and her grandparents. Who were my mother's aunts and uncles and what had happened to them? Where else in her family had this disease ravaged minds and destroyed lives? The search to find the answers obsessed me.

I went through records in libraries, in colleges, in run-down court houses, and in dusty city-hall archives. I walked through old cemeteries, reading the names on the headstones. Finally, I found where my grandmother had been buried. She was listed under the name Hayles, J. F. (Mrs.) in the Oakwood Cemetery in Montgomery, Alabama. She died in 1899, and was buried in Burial lot 4, Square 14, Survey 3.

The record stated that she was twenty-seven years old, white, female. No first name was cited. She lived and died without an identity of her own. The death certificate listed dysentery and miscarriage as the cause of death. There was no record of John F. Hayles in that Alabama Cemetery. I could find no other records of her family anywhere. We will never know if she was the carrier. At twenty-seven, whatever secrets her body may have held about Alzheimer's disease were buried with her.

Perhaps one of her brothers or sisters was afflicted. Susie had one full sister, Amy, and one full brother, Herman. Amy died in her mid-eighties. Her mind was sharp and clear until she died. Herman was what they called a "blue baby," meaning that the umbilical cord was caught around his neck, preventing oxygen from getting to the brain. He was mentally retarded, lived in the county home, and died in a fire accident when he was in his late fifties. Susie's half-sisters were named Corinne, Minnie Kate, and Ruth. Minnie Kate died in childbirth when she was thirty. Did she carry the dreaded gene? Had she lived, would this insidious killer have taken her life? Her children are not effected. Are they carrying a hidden killer lying in wait to strike innocent, future generations? Corinne and Ruth are still living. Corinne is in her nineties; Ruth is in her eighties. Their minds remained clear. None of their children have been affected.

Mama had two half-brothers, Frank, who came to her funeral, and John Henry. In his late twenties, John Henry died a mysterious death, and either no one knew much about it, or no one wanted to talk about what they knew. It appeared that he had been murdered, but no one would say for sure. Was John Henry a carrier? Was his early death a twisted blessing? Frank was never seen again after Mama's funeral. He was forty-seven at the time. Could it be that he developed the disease later than his sister had, and unable to contact any of his family, had died of Alzheimer's disease without any of us knowing it? All are frivolous questions that have no answers.

Perhaps the disease came from my grandfather's family. What about his parents, his grandparents, his brothers and sisters, his aunts and uncles? Corinne,

Mama's half sister, was cooperative and helpful. We
talked many times on the phone. She sent me a family
history written in 1877 by her father, John F. Hayles,
long before he met and married my grandmother,
Minnie Webb. What struck me about my grandfather's
story was the inordinate number of early deaths. He
named person after person, brothers, sisters, aunts,
uncles and cousins, who had died in early childhood
or in their teens or as young adults, too early to have
been hit by Alzheimer's disease, if indeed the dreaded
disease would have struck any of them had they lived.

My grandfather himself was orphaned at an
early age. When he was ten, his mother and father died
within six months of each other during a flu epidemic.
I could find nothing more about his parents. I wonder
if they carried the dreaded gene that would have led
to deaths more cruel than the ones that took their young
lives. Can one person carry this hidden killer, and while
not being affected, harbor the gene to pass on to children or grandchildren yet unborn? How many generations could be skipped, only to have the killer gene
emerge and wield its deadly terror once again? Where
does it lie hidden in my family? I was filled with haunting questions and was finding no answers. The hundreds of hours spent in dusty towns going through
old records yielded no significant information.

Discouraged at finding no clear family pattern
to share with the researchers, I was determined to do
what I could with the information we had on our own
family. When Johnny and I first broached the subject

of being tested, some family members hesitated. It is an understandable reluctance. Who wants to have confirmed the possibility that this tragic and dreadful disease loomed in their futures? Denial is easier and less painful and is a strong protector against frightening and unwanted knowledge. It is easy to think that, if we don't acknowledge something, maybe it won't happen.

Becoming involved in the research project on familial Alzheimer's disease would make real the possibility that any one of us could be next. But after much discussion on the value of research, coupled with the fact that the researchers would come to them to draw blood, one by one, members of the family courageously agreed. It was all terribly frightening. They would participate perhaps for themselves, but more likely, they would become involved in this research for their children and their grandchildren, and for all people who would suffer from Alzheimer's disease. Today, they are willing participants whenever they are called upon to help.

I have been tested regularly since the early eighties and have been involved in research projects in the University of Colorado School of Medicine in Denver, at the Veteran's Hospital in Palo Alto, California, at the University of Washington School of Medicine, Department of Medical Genetics, and the Alzheimer's Disease Research Center in Washington State, and the Alzheimer's Disease Research Center in Tulsa, Oklahoma, at the Veteran's Hospital in conjunction with

UCLA Medical School, and at the University of San Diego.

Today, the Veteran's Hospital in Palo Alto, California, has a unit dedicated to Alzheimer's disease research patients and their families. This unit has private bathrooms, televisions, and all the extras. When I first went for tests, and they wanted to do several days of testing, they didn't have a place for me to stay over night. I ended up in the room where they did sleep studies.

Whenever I left the room, the door locked automatically, so I had to prop the door open when I left the bed during the night to use the bathroom. I would dash as fast as I could, clutching my errant hospital gown to keep it from flapping open in back and hoping I would not to be locked out in the hall.

I went regularly to the Palo Alto Veteran's Hospital. Shortly after Leonard's death, I was there for testing. Helen Davies, the psychiatric clinical nurse doing the testing, noticed something was wrong. She didn't want to continue the testing until she found out what was troubling me. She kept asking me what was the matter. I kept telling her that there was nothing the matter. It was clear that she didn't believe me. Finally, she asked if Leonard had died recently. I told her that, yes, he had.

"Have you grieved?" she asked kindly.

"No," I answered firmly. "I'll not shed another tear over Alzheimer's. Not one more tear. I've cried all

I am ever going to cry over what it's done to my family. I am finished grieving. I'm through with it." As I finished blurting out my response to her, I was shrieking, my voice having given way to anger.

"It's normal to grieve when someone dies," she said gently.

"No," I repeated. "I'm all through grieving. I will not grieve anymore. Not ever again. Never." I spoke passionately, convinced that my grieving was over and trying to convince Helen Davies of my conviction.

She tried a while longer to encourage me to acknowledge my grief. I wouldn't budge from my position. When she saw that she wasn't making any progress, she called the head psychologist, Dr. Jared Tinklenberg. Both of them talked and talked to me about my need to grieve, and finally I began to cry. Next thing I knew, I was crying like a lost child, sobbing uncontrollably. I stayed at the hospital and cried continually for two days and two nights. My face was so swollen, I could hardly open my eyes. On the third day, I stopped crying, and Helen Davies administered the tests without a hitch. This experience taught me the importance of grieving. It has helped me help others go through the grieving process.

I have had CAT scans, MRI's, and PET scans. I have donated blood, urine, skin, and saliva. I have taken more psychological tests than I care to remember. And yes, I know who the President of the United States is!

As of the writing of this book, they say that I am fine. Perfectly normal. Johnny kids me and says he wants a second opinion. He says that he is willing to donate my brain to science, but the doctors insist that he'll have to wait until I am dead. Johnny never lets me get too serious when I start worrying about how the tests might come out. So far, I'm fine, and since I am now sixty, I am past the age for the type of Alzheimer's disease that struck my family. Now, I have the same chance as anybody else has. Today, I am no longer afraid for myself. I still harbor fears for my children and grandchildren and pray that this horror will never enter their lives.

When we first asked the family about being tested, Anna June was working at a job where she didn't want anyone to know that there was Alzheimer's disease in her family. Later, she agreed to participate. It took a great deal of courage. I admire my sister.

My sister, Minnie Sue, was deteriorating rapidly, and I felt an intense urge to travel to Kansas City to see her. Knowing how I had reacted to previous visits to my ill relatives, my family and friends strongly counseled me not to go.

"There's no way she's going to even recognize you, Bea, so what's the point of going?"

"It's a waste of time and money, and you'll only just get yourself all upset. Why on earth do you want to put yourself through all of that? Bea, be reasonable."

"You know how emotional you are, Bea. We'll end up having to put you in the hospital, too. Use your head and don't go. It would be foolish for you to make this trip. Think about what it does to your family, Bea."

But Johnny supported me as he always does. He told me, "Bea, you do what you feel you have to do." I knew I had to make this trip.

When I arrived at the nursing home, I found my sister Minnie Sue as limp as a rag and tied in a wheel chair. I knew that if she had not been tied, she would have slid to the floor. Her head hung to one side. Drool ran from the corner of her mouth. I was struck by her appearance. She looked just like Mama. It was a heart wrenching, emotional visit, but this time, for the first time, I didn't fall apart. I didn't become hysterical.

I approached my sister, placed my hand on her shoulder, and gently brushed her cheek with my finger. Then I carefully lifted her face so that she could see me and I spoke to her softly,

"Minnie Sue, this is Bea. I am Bea, your little sister. I love you, Minnie Sue, and I've come to see you. Minnie Sue, I am your little sister, Bea."

Minnie Sue looked up at me. Her eyes were expressionless as they found my face. She repeated plaintively, "Mama. Mama." That was all she said, and then she cried. From somewhere deep within her, a sadness found expression. I cried with her, not in desperation as I had before, but in compassion and love for my sister. I hoped that she had at least recognized me as someone in her family who cared. And then again, maybe "Mama" was the only word she knew how to say any more. I will never know. I chose to believe that she recognized me as someone in her family who loved her, and that alone made the trip worthwhile. I thanked God that I had come.

This time the return trip from Kansas City was different for me, too. I knew now that I must do something. A commitment to take some kind of action was growing in me. After seeing Herschel in the final throes of this cruel disease, I was a basket case for weeks, sometimes crying hysterically in fear that my turn would soon come. Not this time. I still knew that I might well be next, but I had changed. Knowing that my Lord was always with me gave me serenity and strength. This time, when Johnny met me at the airport, I was bursting to share my feelings and determination with him.

"My God, Johnny, we have to do something or this disease will wipe us all out. I must do something," I told him.

"Good," he responded, and then asked, "What do you have in mind?"

I paused, not sure quite what to say. I had formulated no plan.

"Nothing yet," I answered. "I don't know what I'll do, and I don't have the slightest idea where to begin, but I am absolutely positive that I must do something. And, Johnny, I know that I will do something," I said with conviction and determination. He patted my shoulder reassuringly, and we walked to the car in silence.

My first step was to talk to my doctor who suggested that I see a neurologist. I made an appointment. I set out to educate myself by learning more about Alzheimer's disease from an expert who really understood the disease. I sat in this learned doctor's office and explained why I had come. He appeared somewhat impatient as he swiveled his chair around and took a book from the hundreds of volumes on the shelves behind him. He flipped through the pages, and then read a one sentence definition of Alzheimer's disease. He closed the book and replaced it.

"That's all I can tell you," he said, shrugging his shoulders.

I felt as though someone had slapped me. My disappointment must have been apparent, because the doctor got out of his chair, walked to the door, and opened it for me. His actions were a clear but wordless invitation for me to leave. As I walked out of his office, the woman at the front desk said, "That will be thirty-five dollars, please."

Once outside, I explained to my husband what had happened and said incredulously, "You know, Johnny, I believe that I know more about the disease than that doctor does."

"Yes, I'm afraid you do," Johnny responded.

He was right. It was a discouraging first step on my journey to save the suffering.

My day-to-day life in Tahoe continued. I worked at several different jobs. One of them was as a sales clerk in a dress shop. I rather liked working there where

I sold nice clothes and met lovely people. One woman I met while I was working there had worked at the Mayo Clinic. She suggested that I write to the major research hospitals to find out what information they might have. I was reluctant at first, questioning how a woman with a marginal, ninth-grade education could write to such prestigious places, but I decided to write anyway. In October of 1975, I began the second step of my journey.

I was surprised and delighted to receive an answer. A letter dated October 28, 1975, arrived from Dr. Robert C. Hermann. The contents were not encouraging.

> Alzheimer's disease is a disease which is usually not inherited, but on occasion it does run in families. In those families, it is hard to determine what the mode of inheritance is; and for that reason, it is difficult to be sure what your children's chances of getting it would be. Whenever we see patients with similar diseases in a family, we often wonder if the diagnosis is correct. If, indeed, this illness is Alzheimer's disease, there is no known method of prevention and no known method of early diagnosis that would benefit your children or yourself that I am aware of.

He thanked me for my letter and suggested that if I sent more information, perhaps he could be of more help. I didn't have any more information. Although he questioned the accuracy of the diagnosis of Alzheimer's disease, at least he had taken the time to answer my letter. Instead of feeling discouraged, I was encouraged and emboldened by the response. I went to the library and checked out a reference book which listed all the university hospitals in the United States and their addresses and began writing letters in earnest.

Most responses parroted the Mayo Clinic's response. Some were much less kind. A few said quite bluntly that I probably didn't know what I was talking about, since Alzheimer's disease does not run in families and is a very rare disease. They questioned whether or not the diagnoses of my mother and brothers and sisters were accurate.

They consistently explained that little was known about Alzheimer's and that the disease was very rare. Some letters were condescending and others were downright rude. One doctor explained that he wouldn't be able to explain it to me in a way that I could understand it. I figured he probably couldn't explain it because he didn't know very much about it to explain. I must say that all of my letter writing took place in the seventies when, indeed, little was known about Alzheimer's disease. Whatever the reasons, I obviously wasn't setting the medical world on fire with my information about my family. Not one of them was

the least bit intrigued by my story nor by my commitment to find out what I could do to protect my children and nieces and nephews, as well as myself and
my remaining sisters.

For some reason, I had neglected to write to the
University of Colorado in Denver. A visiting friend
encouraged me to write them. That letter resulted in
one of the most precious pieces of mail I have ever received. In a letter dated December 2, 1975, James Austin, M.D., Professor and Chair of the Department of
Neurology at the University of Colorado Medical
School said,

"Not only are we doing research on Alzheimer's
disease we are doing research on Familial Alzheimer's
disease.... It may be that some of the studies we could
offer you might be of some help in finding out whether
or not you might be at risk."

In his letter, Dr. Austin invited me to come to
Denver. Would I please call him? Letter in hand, I ran
around the house like some kind of nut, waving the
letter in the air and shouting at the top of my lungs to
an empty house, "Somebody out there cares! Somebody out there wants to do something! Somebody listened! They care! Oh, thank God. Thank you, thank
you, dear God."

I couldn't contain my excitement. I was laughing and crying at the same time. Had anyone witnessed
my jumping and running around the house, or heard
my whooping and squealing, I'm sure they would have
suspected the worst.

I was eager to go to Denver, but it wasn't until about six months later that Johnny and I could make the trip. Going through papers, I gathered every scrap I had collected, including my "family tree" and stuffed it into a brown envelope. It looked very much like a pile of trash. Packed and ready, Johnny and I drove to Colorado. He stayed with his parents while I checked into the hospital.

Upon arrival, I presented my mishmash collection of information to the researchers, and they copied every piece as though they'd found a treasure. When they gave my pile of papers back to me in a new envelope, it was labeled, "Bea's Manuscript." How good it felt to feel valued. Here I was not ridiculed. I had something important to share, and they knew it, and they appreciated it. My journey was looking up. My efforts had paid off. As the Bible says, "Seek and ye shall find."

While in Denver, Dr. Austin told me he was studying two families, including our family, who had Familial Alzheimer's disease. He mentioned a family being studied by Daniel A. Pollen, M.D., Professor of Neurology and Physiology at the University of Massachusetts Medical Center. This family had emigrated from Eastern Europe. The mother, Hannah, had Alzheimer's disease, and four of her nine children developed Alzheimer's disease. They had records of four generations. A chill ran through me. My mother Susie had Alzheimer's disease, and four of her nine children developed the Alzheimer's disease. What information would four generations of our family yield?

The family being studied at the University of Colorado in Denver had thirteen out of fourteen children who had developed the disease. Today, many families are being studied, but ours was one of the first. It was rewarding to me to be a primary part of this crucial research. I was determined to do all I possibly could to help.

Over a three day period, I went through every test imaginable. I had just turned forty at the time, and although I was coming into the danger years, I didn't panic. The CAT Scan showed no problems. Psychological tests indicated no characteristics exhibited by early stage Alzheimer's patients, but the doctors gently told me that they could give me no guarantees. At least I wasn't showing any signs of being in the early stages of the disease. Still, the doctors indicated that it was like tossing a coin. It could go either way. Miraculously, I did not panic or become discouraged.

A young intern, who didn't look over seventeen or eighteen, did most of the testing. In spite of his boyish appearance, his commitment and competence were of someone far beyond his years. His name is Bob Cook-Deegan, M.D., and he helped our family become involved in research and our new organization by speaking to one of our first support groups.

Doctor Bob ask me if there were things our family did that were different from what most families did. He wanted to know if the ones who had Alzheimer's disease have any behaviors in common. I told him that since we were poor, and we had nine hungry kids, we ate lots of beans. I didn't know if other families who ate lots of beans had these problems. I also explained that Mama never smoked, drank or cussed, but my brothers did all of these things. At least in our family, there didn't seem to be any relationship between what a person did or ate and who got sick.

It was through the researchers at the University of Colorado that I received a letter from Dr. Ben Williamson, himself a member of a family decimated by the disease. Dr. Williamson was the Miners' mentor and the one who persuaded them to study familial Alzheimer's disease. He told Dr. Gary Miner and Dr. Linda Winters-Miner about our family.

When Gary Miner and I first spoke on the phone, it was like a heavenly designed appointment. He came to California to test members of my family, and later, I flew to Boston to present my story at a support group and to be tested again. The Miners have played a key role in my efforts to do something to help victims and caregivers. Gary and Linda Miner started their work in 1973, when few people had even heard of Alzheimer's disease, let alone familial Alzheimer's disease. They were pioneers. It took courage to speak out at a time when the idea that Alzheimer's disease ran in families was being ridiculed by mainstream thinking. Today, the gene has been found that causes the type of Alzheimer's disease that is inherited!

In 1977, the Miners organized the First International Symposium on Familial Alzheimer's Disease. Scientists came from all over the world. From France,

Germany, Australia, Italy, England, Harvard University , the University of Washington in Seattle, and the National Institute of Health. The first scientific book about how this disease ran in families was written as a result of this conference. Dr. Miner has spoken at our workshops and to our support groups. He and his wife have been an inspiration to me.

Together they founded the Familial Alzheimer's Disease Research Foundation, called the Alzheimer's Foundation, in Tulsa, Oklahoma, and worked tirelessly and in a mission-driven fashion to get the scientists of the world interested in familial Alzheimer's disease. Their work resulted in a book for caregivers called *Caring for Alzheimer's Patients*. Medical research and thinking about familial Alzheimer's disease has come a long way since I first met the Miners. I'll always remember the comfort it gave me to have these highly respected people believe the disease ran in families and dedicate themselves to researching familial Alzheimer's disease.

It was through the Miners that I met Dr. Thomas Bird, a medical researcher from the University of Washington, Department of Neurology and Medical Genetics. We were at a conference in Oklahoma where I had been asked to tell my story. After it was over, Dr. Bird offered to drive me to the airport, since we were both flying out. The long drive plus a delayed flight gave us the opportunity to talk. He asked if he could include our family in his research on Alzheimer's disease being done at the VA Medical Center and University of Washington. I eagerly became involved and asked members of my family if they would also participate. All of them agreed.

My trip to Denver opened many doors and was fruitful in many ways. Dr. Bob gave me the name of the wife of one of the victims of the family where thirteen of fourteen had the disease. I would have traveled to the ends of the earth to find someone else who had gone through what my family was going through, somebody to talk to who would understand.

Her name is Esther Reiswig, and she lived in Oklahoma. I set out to find her. My efforts were futile until I asked my brother-in-law for help. He was in the service, and by strange coincidence, was stationed in this same town in Oklahoma. He simply called the local sheriff, who called her on her CB car radio. The lady I was searching for called me within minutes.

My years of feeling so terribly isolated were over. We hit it off immediately and would talk often on the phone, usually after eleven at night when the rates were lower. It's a good thing we called late, because as it was, our phone bills were out of sight. We developed a friendship that has lasted over the years. She has come to visit us, and I have been to her home. The minute we get together, we talk nonstop. Feelings of validation come from talking with someone who genuinely understands. Finding Esther was a thrilling experience for me.

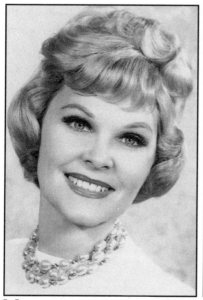

Mary

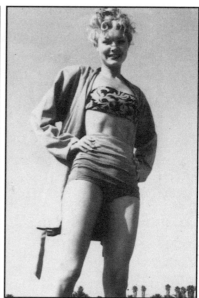

Tommy Lou

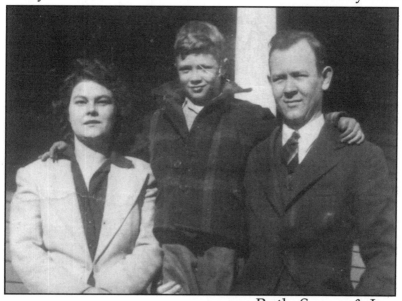

Ruth, Sonny, & Joe

CHAPTER TEN

Minnie Sue

Minnie Sue married when I was five, so again, I don't remember much about her living at home. When I was grown and married, Johnny and had I moved west, so I wasn't around when she was ill with Alzheimer's disease. Her daughter, Anna Sue, shared what she knew with us.

Minnie and her husband Frank divorced when Anna Sue was about a year old. Minnie had a job in a large bank. She enjoyed her work and had no desire to change. Anna Sue felt that if her mother had made the effort, she could have gotten a better job or at least advanced in the one she had, and the two of them could have lived better. As it was, even though Minnie Sue had a regular job, they struggled to make ends meet.

Her reluctance to change jobs could also have been due to her fear that something was wrong. She may have been exhibiting some early signs of the onset of Alzheimer's disease, making advancement out of the question. There is no way of knowing for sure.

Minnie Sue remarried a much older man named Ed. Now I had two brothers-in-law named Ed. He was good to her and stood by her until she died. Ruth and Anna June also helped care for Minnie Sue.

Around 1962, when Minnie Sue was in her early forties, the symptoms became obvious. She would hallucinate and dream up things that had never happened. She would imagine seeing and hearing things that were never there. In 1966, she was in an auto accident, and as a result, pulled some ligaments in her hands. She took a leave of absence from her job and never returned to work. She had held a reasonably responsible job running an IBM machine at a bank in Kansas City.

We found out later that Minnie Sue had been having many problems at work. She would recognize errors and then would forget to correct them. She would make errors and not recognize them. She would forget what she was supposed to be doing. Sometimes, she would leave her desk to do something, forget what she had set out to do, become side tracked, and not return to her work station for an hour or more. She would forget to show up for work.

Always in the past, Minnie Sue had been very professional and prided herself in being well dressed and well groomed. Now she was dressing carelessly, wearing clothes that didn't go together or weren't clean or pressed, shoes that weren't appropriate for the office, blouses over dresses, or other mismatched accumulations of garments. She would forget that she had eaten and eat again. Although her weight had not varied during her first forty years, she promptly gained thirty-five or forty pounds. Her clothes no longer fit properly and would gap where they couldn't be buttoned or zipped, or would be pinned awkwardly.

Anna Sue asked her mother one day if she thought perhaps she had the same thing that her mother Susie had. Minnie Sue's response was immediate and definite.

"Oh, no. I just have nerves, and I'm probably going through the change."

Minnie Sue often would become lost and would always call Ruth, our oldest sister and the one very close to Minnie Sue, to come get her and take her home. When she could no longer find her way, she stopped going out of the house and would pass the time continually cleaning and by putting pictures in photo albums. She would clean the same room over and over again, mopping an already-scrubbed floor or vacuuming a spotless carpet. She would put pictures in the album and take them out, put them back in, and then remove them again. More and more of the pictures would be placed in the album up-side-down, but Minnie Sue didn't seem to notice.

Unlike Herschel, Minnie did not find her reflection in the mirror to be friendly and was frightened by the total stranger she saw. Eventually, Minnie Sue would become so frightened, she would be hysterical, and her husband, Ed, had to cover or remove all the mirrors in the home.

As she deteriorated, she would sit for hours and watch TV. She never spoke of her past, never mentioned her mother or father. Her speech was the first to go, and in her frustration of not being able to talk, she would often strike out and hit people. Ruth told us that Minnie Sue often attempted to hit her. Minnie Sue loved Ruth and would never have struck her sister if she hadn't been ill.

Unable to speak, she swore in frustration. Minnie Sue had not been one to use colorful language, but now she would just sit and say, "Shit!" over and over. That's all she would say.

She also became incontinent right away. This is usually one of the last things that happens. Ed had to change her diapers. Minnie Sue was still having her period, making Ed's job more difficult.

Until the final stages, Minnie Sue was able to be cared for at home. She was soon unable to feed herself. Ruth and Anna Sue changed her and fed her. When she fainted at home one day, it was clear to them that she needed to be where she would have twenty-four-hour care, so she was placed in a convalescent hospital. In 1974, after a year there, she passed away. She was fifty-three.

Ruth was the first to realize that Minnie Sue had her Mama's disease, but she hesitated to share what she knew with the rest of the family. She didn't want to frighten everybody. She also didn't want to believe it herself. By not saying anything, she didn't have to deal with the family's reaction to having another one of us being struck down by Alzheimer's disease. Until it was obvious to everyone, Ruth didn't say anything.

CHAPTER ELEVEN

The Alzheimer's Aid Society

I was working as a receptionist for the *Lake Tahoe News*, a small local newspaper, when Esther called to tell me that a woman named Bobbie Glaze from Edina, Minnesota, had been organizing and facilitating support groups. She was the first person to do something about helping people who lived with and took care of Alzheimer's patients. Mrs. Glaze's husband had Alzheimer's disease, and she knew what people like us were going through. At first, the groups were for caregivers of people who had mental illness of any kind. Later, she organized support groups for caregivers of victims of Alzheimer's disease. At last, people who lived with Alzheimer's patients would have a chance to meet and share their experiences. A large support group was scheduled to be held in Denver, Colorado, and the another one would be held in San Diego, California.

Money was tight, but I knew I had to attend. In July of 1980, Wendy, my youngest daughter, and her four-month-old son Joshua, went with me to Denver. Wendy had just lost her husband, and I thought taking this trip might be good for her.

That first support group meeting made a profound impression on me. It is difficult for me to explain the connection a person has with others who have suffered the same pain, ached from the same guilt, or wept in the same frustrations and feelings of helplessness. These people had spent their share of sleepless nights in fear, not only of what was happening to their loved ones, but of what might happen to them. Everyone in this room had a person in their family who suffered from Alzheimer's disease. I was not the only one who had felt so terribly alone. There were people all around me who had felt the same way.

When I returned to Lake Tahoe, I talked with the editor of the paper and told her about my trip and my family history. She thought my story would make an interesting article for the paper. Jim Sloan, a reporter for the paper, interviewed me, and on August 2, 1980, his article, "Family Battles Unknown Killer," appeared in the *Lake Tahoe News*. That was the first time my story was told publicly. As a result of that article, a woman came into the office and asked for Bea Gorman. Her husband had been diagnosed with Alzheimer's disease. He was forty-eight years old, and they had a son who was not quite two. The diagnosis was devastating to her. She was eager to learn more about the disease and to help others in any way she could. She was young and bright and full of energy. Her name was Margie.

The two of us met frequently and talked end-lessly about our plights. I shared what I could to help her deal with what she was facing. We discussed how we might organize to help others. We had originally thought that we would have our first support group in Tahoe or Reno. We decided on the name for our or-ganization, The Alzheimer's Aid Society. I was presi-dent. She was vice president.

We entered a parade in Placerville to let people know about what we were doing. We drove a van and had a banner with large letters draped across the side announcing the Alzheimer's Aid Society. People were so frightened, they didn't want to come near the van. They were afraid of catching the disease. If we were going to educate the public about Alzheimer's disease, we had our work cut out for us.

Margie was the only one who responded to the Tahoe article. Then Jim Sloan sold his article to the *Sacramento Bee*. At the end of the article was a note to write to Bea Gorman at *The Lake Tahoe News* if anyone wanted more information. Calls and letters started pouring in from all over Northern California. Most of them were from the Sacramento area. They didn't ask if we were going to start a support group. They wanted to know when and where we were starting a support group. We decided that Sacramento was the logical place to begin, and that it was time we got started.

Margie was a doer. I was still working full time and had four kids. Margie had a young child and a sick husband, but still, her time was more flexible than

mine. Of the two of us, she was definitely the orga-
nizer.

After many phone calls and letters to the people
who had responded to *The Sacramento Bee* article,
Margie and I held our first support group meeting in
Sacramento on March 6, 1981. Seventy-five people
showed up. I started the meeting by telling the story
of my mother, my brothers and sisters. One by one,
others began to share, but because the group was so
large, not everybody had a chance to talk. We passed
around a sign-up sheet. That was the beginning of our
mailing list. We told everybody that we would let them
know when the next meeting was scheduled. The
Alzheimer's Aid Society was off and running.

One of the letters in response to the article in
The Sacramento Bee asked if I would be willing to appear on a radio talk show. I agreed. That was my first
time on radio. More calls and letters arrived in response
to the radio show.

The letters arriving day after day touched me
deeply and were an inspiration to me. People were
desperate for help and information. It is difficult for
me to describe the urgency expressed by these letters.
I want to share one with you.

October 23, 1981

Dear Mrs. Gorman,

I don't know how to start this letter. Your article in the Sacramento Bee really touched home with me. It's all I've
been able to think about.

About three years ago, my mother was diagnosed as having Alzheimer's. This was the first time I or my family had heard of the disease. My mother is now in a mental hospital doing very poorly. I don't know how to tell you what it feels like to watch someone you love go through this.

Mrs. Gorman, I am also frightened. I am twenty-eight-years old and have two small children. Although my mother is the first victim of this disease in our family, at least that I know of, I am worried for myself, my kids, and my sisters. We were told Alzheimer's was rare and not much else.

If you could find the time, I would like to know more about the testing you had at the University of Colorado. I'm not sure I would have the courage to have the testing. I only wish this disease was not so hopeless.

Thank you so much for coming forward and sharing such a painful part of your life. I hope you receive a lot of response and help in your crusade. Please contact me if I can do anything to help. Thank you again.

People knew so little about Alzheimer's disease and were desperate to learn more. People felt alone. They wanted to help and be helped. Letters like this one, and there were many, made me more committed than ever to help in any way I could.

On April 10, 1981, Margie and I held our second support group meeting in a large church in West Sacramento. Bob Cook-Deegan, M.D., the neurologist doing research at the University of Colorado who had been so helpful to me when I was being tested was coming out to gather blood samples from members of my family. While he was here, he readily agreed to speak to our group. Johnny had contacted Pierre Dreyfus, M.D., Professor and Chair of the Department of Neurology at the University of California, Davis. He also agreed to speak. We were excited to have such important presenters for our fledgling organization.

Ed drove Norma Jean up from Los Angeles so that she could participate in the testing. He has always been eager and cooperative to do whatever he could to help. They stayed in town to attend our support group meeting.

We decided to hold regular meetings on the second Friday of each month. Margie and I would drive down from Lake Tahoe and stay in a motel. We began gathering printed information on Alzheimer's disease and distributing it to the group.

Joan Sahl, a geriatric nurse from Roseville, asked if she could coordinate a group in her area and still rely on us for information and support. That was how our second support group was started. People living nearer to Roseville could attend there, which allowed the Sacramento group to settle into a more manageable size. Then a request came to begin a group in Auburn, and the Alzheimer's Aid Society now offered support groups in three locations. We were growing.

Today there are twenty-six groups in our network of organizations. We have had as many as thirty. The Alzheimer's Aid Society, supplies support to these groups at no charge. We have no dues for membership. We speak to their groups and help them line up other speakers. We supply printed information and the free use of videos and other program materials. Each group sends us their membership list and receives our bimonthly newsletter.

We help in finding group facilitators if they need us to do that. Often a professional in the field will volunteer to facilitate. That lead person is crucial. The most important thing, other than having experience with Alzheimer's, is that the person is a caring person. We have been so fortunate that so many good, caring people have come forward to volunteer.

After those initial meetings, sometimes we had a speaker and sometimes we showed a video, but mostly, people came to the group to talk about their lives and their struggles in dealing with Alzheimer's disease. They needed to share the pain and frustration. They gathered ideas of things to do that might help. A strong camaraderie existed in these support groups.

Seventy-five people in a group are far too many if people want the chance to share. People who come to support groups need to talk. They spend most of their time with a person who has Alzheimer's disease where normal conversation is impossible. They come to share and to find support. We soon learned that groups should have no more than fifteen or twenty people in them to be effective. With too many in a group, it's impossible for everyone to have a chance to talk. Talking is important.

After about a year of holding regular meetings, Johnny and I took a long-planned vacation. While we were gone, and without saying anything to me, Margie and another woman, who had been attending the support group meetings, decided it would be better to form their own separate organization. Margie was a natural leader and very capable. I can see now why she didn't think she needed to include me. She was confident that she and this new woman could do more and move faster than she and I could.

Margie wrote or called everyone on our list inviting them to join the new group with her. Now that's a perfectly fine thing to want to do, but when they set up a meeting in the same building and intercepted people coming in and directed them to the meeting she was holding without letting me know, I was devastated. I didn't have a clue that anything like this was going on. I found out when my sister Tommy Lou was coming to our meeting and was intercepted in the hall and told not to go our meeting, but to go to the one down the hall instead.

I was so hurt. I wanted to give up. The depression I felt paralyzed me. I couldn't understand why she would do this. I was always very comfortable being in the background, but I didn't want to be left out completely! I was so naive. I took it personally. It didn't occur to me that maybe she thought that she could do more with this new group. This new group, however, never did get off the ground and eventually folded.

Today, I am very grateful to her for the work she did. Today, I know that thousands of people need help, and there is room for anybody who wants to volunteer. There is room for as many groups as possible. At the time, though, I just felt betrayed. I felt rejected. It would have been better if she had said something to me, but that wasn't the way it worked out.

Anyway, I was ready to quit. My feelings were so hurt that I just wanted to crawl in a hole and lick my wounds. This time Johnny didn't support me. He didn't say, "You do what you think you have to do, Bea," like he usually did. He didn't like my wanting to jump ship. He told me that people needed what I was doing and that I should stick with it. He told me that what I was doing was important. Lots more important than a few hurt feelings. Johnny wasn't about to let me quit.

Johnny was working long hours, but he still took time to help me. Without fail, he went with me to the support group meetings in Sacramento. Still, it was up to me to hold the group together and do all the preparation and follow-up work. For the first time in my

life, I didn't have anyone to lean on. I didn't have anyone to follow. I had to lead. It was frightening. I wasn't
sure if I could continue.

I was still thinking about quitting and had pretty
much made up my mind to do just that. I'm a quitter, I
guess. I hate unpleasantness and confrontation. I just
can't bear it. I was afraid of stepping out on my own to
run the Alzheimer's Aid Society. I went ahead with
the bake sale because we had already planned to hold
it in order to raise money for our organization, but I
had made up my mind that this would be the last thing
I would do. I would quit at the end of the day. So much
for my commitment to helping people cope with
Alzheimer's disease. I was afraid and feeling sorry for
myself big time!

At the bake sale, an elderly woman on one crutch
kept walking back and forth and back and forth in front
of our table. After awhile, she slowly hobbled up to
me, and, with tears in her eyes, thanked me for doing
what we were doing.

"You just don't know how much this helps me,
seeing you here," she said. "I was just diagnosed with
Alzheimer's. I didn't think that there was anybody out
there who knew anything about it. This means so much
to me to know you're out there and you care. Somebody cares." Tears streamed down her cheeks.

That little lady turned me around. She inspired
me. How dare I be a quitter? After all, if I was doing
this because I wanted to help people, here was someone who needed my help. Here was a person grateful

for what I was doing. I knew then that I couldn't quit. The woman's name was Donna Hayes, and she became our friend, and for years, as long as she was able to attend, Johnny and I picked her up and took her to our support group meetings. Later, I felt that Donna Hayes was a message from the Lord telling me not to give up, telling me that I had a job to do.

Anyway, with Johnny telling me not to quit and willing to help me, and with this dear lady thanking me for helping, I hung in there. Rain, flash floods, snow, road detours, it didn't matter. Once a month, Johnny and I drove to Sacramento for the support group meeting. If the group had too many people in it to allow time for everyone to talk, we broke up into two groups. I took one, and Johnny took the other. He had learned a great deal through his experiences in dealing with my family, but now he began study in earnest. He read everything he could get his hands on. He listened with renewed interest to the stories being shared.

During this time, I attended a conference held at Stanford University. One of the speakers was George Glenner, M.D., Professor of Pathology at the University of California, San Diego, School of Medicine, and one of the world's leading researchers on Alzheimer's disease. He was also one of the most caring and dedicated men I have ever known. Our family participated in the research he was doing. Again and again, Dr. Glenner gave generously of his time and wisdom. He spoke to our workshops and to our support groups. He and his wife Joy founded a series of day care centers for Alzheimer's patients. Joy Glenner directed the centers and is known, not just for her extensive knowledge, but for her compassion for those who suffer from this mind twisting disease, and for their families, who also suffer. Dr. Glenner passed away just as this book was being finished. He leaves a profound empty place in my heart. Johnny and I will always treasure and remember what the Glenners have done for us.

Attending conferences and workshops helped me to know and understand more about the disease that consumed my life and put me in contact with a network of others dedicated to searching for a cure or to helping victims, caregivers, and families. In the meantime, I also took classes on computers and office management at the community college in Lake Tahoe. It was a wonderful new world for me. I loved it. Spring rain or winter snow, it didn't matter, I was there, usually arriving well before class started. I was like a sponge. I couldn't get enough information. My instructors loved my eagerness and always went the extra mile to give me more information. College courses were a far cry from the boredom and alienation I felt in high school.

The Alzheimer's Aid Society was growing. More and more satellite groups started. We have never gone out to start groups. People have always come to us. We provide literature free of charge, except for books. We provide copies of literature at no cost for distribution to support group attendees and anyone else who wants to learn more about Alzheimer's disease. We lend videos and books. We do not charge for any of the services we provide, but we do take donations. People have been very generous to our organization.

Calls continued to come in asking me to speak to groups throughout Northern California. More and more articles appeared in local papers resulting in more calls. Letters continued to pour in. I was on television and radio again and again. I told my story over and over.

There was one major problem. Speaking shredded me emotionally. Each time I spoke, it was as though I had to live through all of the pain again. Going over and over the pain of my family and how this horrible illness took away their dignity took its toll on me. I would be exhausted for days. I didn't enjoy getting up in front of people. In fact, I dreaded it, but I forced myself to continue. For about ten years, I did all of the speaking. Just when I felt that I could not go on, Johnny retired and became much more active in the Alzheimer's Aid Society. Not only is he an excellent speaker, he is knowledgeable, and he enjoys speaking to groups.

Today, Johnny does all the speaking, the training sessions, and public relations work for us. I organize the work done at the office, facilitate support groups, provide support to families in person and on the phone, as well as organize the workshops and get our newsletter printed and sent out. It is a much better arrangement for me.

Our network of support groups continues to grow. Some groups have been active for years. Others have faded out as the Alzheimer's patients died and caregivers went on with their lives and left the trauma of the disease behind them.

Whenever we are traveling in a new area, we try to visit an Alzheimer's support group. We were visiting a group in San Francisco where we met Dr. Cross, a neurologist. Her presentation was very helpful, so we asked her if she would come to Sacramento and talk to our support group sometime. She told us she would be happy to come. Not only did she drive to Sacramento to speak to our group, she brought her husband, Dr. Robert Friedman, with her. It turned out that he is also a neurologist and one of the leading researchers in the field. We were such novices that we had never heard of him. We soon learned of his reputation. He volunteered to serve as our medical advisor. We felt blessed.

In building our organization, at times it seemed that we learned everything the hard way. Other times, things just fell into our laps. We were so inexperienced. Many times, what seemed to be a setback was really a blessing in disguise. At times we were terribly discouraged, and other times, we felt that God was by our side.

Margie's new organization scheduled a workshop. When Johnny called to see about helping out and being involved in some way, he was told that they didn't want us to participate. Later, Dr. Weiler, the speaker at that first workshop, became a good friend and a strong supporter of our work and our organization. He was generous to us with donations and spoke at several of our workshops, but at the time, he didn't know us from Adam, and rejected Johnny's offer to help.

As usual, I went through being hurt and feeling rejected and sorry for myself. It upset Johnny too, but when something upsets Johnny, he doesn't mope around like I do. Johnny does something about it. Johnny doesn't like to be told he can't do something, so he said, "To heck with them. We'll conduct our own workshop." I laughed at the idea. Actually, if I am going to be honest about it, I scoffed at the idea.

"Oh, sure," I chided him. "What do we know? Who are we to do a workshop? How do you think we are going to do it? That's a crazy idea!"

I should have known. Johnny is always the optimist. I'm the pessimist. When someone tells Johnny he can't do something, that's all the more reason for him to go ahead and do it. The first thing I knew, our first workshop was organized and ready. It went off without a hitch. We had three speakers. Dr. Friedman spoke on medical and research issues. Debbie Bird, a registered nurse whose father had Alzheimer's, talked to the group about patient care. A psychologist, Craig Johnson, Ph.D. lectured on dealing with grief and guilt. Everyone who attended enjoyed it and said they got a lot out of it and wanted us to do more. Over two hundred people attended. Johnny and I were delighted with the workshop's success. Of course, Johnny saw to it that I ate a little crow for doubting him.

For admission, we asked for a donation of ten dollars per person. We wanted to hold a workshop for caregivers rather than for professionals, and it was important to us that the workshop was affordable. Today, we have about half professionals and half caregivers attending. In 1995, we were still charging ten dollars, but we have had to raise that to twenty-five dollars. Since most workshops charge from one hundred-fifty to three hundred dollars, ours is still a bargain.

If we had been welcomed to participate with the other group's first workshop, we wouldn't have done one on our own. Today, our workshops have people waiting to attend. It's hard to explain sometimes how things work out for us. Nothing was ever really planned. One thing after another just happened. When we found the ball in our laps, we picked it up and ran with it.

CHAPTER TWELVE

Leonard, The Second Son

Both boys were handsome, but Leonard was the taller of the two, and people said that he looked just like Tony Curtis. The girls hounded him to death. He complained a lot, but I think he really loved it. He swaggered and talked macho, but underneath it all, he really wasn't that tough. He was mean to us, though. When I was little, and he was about eleven or twelve, he would get angry at me and Anna June and yell at us to go home and leave him and his friends alone. Pretty normal behavior for a boy who didn't want his little sisters pestering him, I guess, but it hurt my feelings nonetheless.

At the top of the stairs there was a closet, and Leonard took it over as his private space. I remember that he collected keys, and the walls were lined with nails with keys hanging on them. None of us littler kids dared go near his hideout.

He, like his brother Herschel, didn't care at all about school work, and dropped out of school to learn

Daddy's trade so he could go to work and earn a living. Leonard was working full time with his daddy and older brother by the time he was fourteen. He was good with his hands and became a highly skilled painter. He, too, hung wall paper and did some carpentry work and plaster repair as needed. Both boys grew up to become competent craftsmen and responsible men. Until their illnesses, they never had trouble finding work.

Leonard's pride and joy was his motorcycle. In spite of all his bravado, I always thought of him as a gentle biker. When Herschel moved to California, Leonard followed him, riding his beloved motorcycle across country. In those days, riders didn't wear helmets and goggles or face shields, and Leonard was badly burned by the sun and wind. He made it to California, though. Soon after he left, his fiancee followed him west, and, on October 6, 1951, Leonard and Evelyn were married. They had three children and lived in California for the rest of their lives.

Johnny and I had not seen Leonard and Evelyn for almost seven years when they showed up unannounced at our front door where we lived near Denver. As adults, we had drifted apart. We were all busy with our own lives and families, so we didn't visit each other very often. It was at a time when Johnny had just bought out his father's share in the meat market and grocery store. Now there was one person doing the work that had been done by two. I was trying to help in any way I could. I'd run errands and things like that. We needed house guests like we needed a hole in the head, but we did our best to be hospitable.

But Leonard was awful. He criticized everything we did. He said that with the way we were raising our kids, our son John Jr., three years old at the time, would end up in trouble. Just what made him think that our little boy would become a delinquent, I don't know, but I was angry. He criticized my housekeeping, which wasn't at its best at the time because we were both working so hard on the store. Still, I didn't need his negative critique. Johnny and I were so proud of the store which was now ours. Leonard had nothing good to say about it, and predicted that it would fall down shortly.

I was devastated and told Leonard and Evelyn that I was leaving to go over to our store, and I wanted them gone when I returned. They left in a huff, and we didn't see them again for years. We didn't consider the possibility that Leonard was obnoxious because he might be exhibiting early symptoms of Alzheimer's disease either.

Leonard's illness came on rather quickly once the symptoms started. His hostile and irresponsible behavior caused his marriage to fall apart. Until the symptoms started, Leonard had been dedicated to his wife and children. Now, he became quite free with his attentions to a variety of women. Leonard and Evelyn divorced in January of 1970. Leonard was forty-two and undoubtedly well into the disease. No one even considered that he might be ill. He was just acting crazy, that was all. Later, Evelyn would regret their breakup because she had no idea that her husband was sick, and that he could not help doing the things he did. Her guilt haunts her to this day.

For awhile, Leonard lived with a woman named Lee, but they never married. Two years after his divorce, when Lee and Leonard were together at Herschel's funeral, they sat apart from the family and giggled and talked through the entire service. People wondered what was wrong. That was the first time any of us admitted to anyone in the family that Leonard might have a problem.

In June of 1974, Leonard remarried again to a woman named Marie. He had just had his forty-sixth birthday. We knew Leonard was having problems, but again, we said nothing. Today, we wonder if Marie would have listened to us had we told her. Love in its early bloom has a way of not listening to sane advice. It is a struggle to know when it is right to step in and when it is better to keep one's counsel. Anyway, we didn't say anything to her.

Leonard forgot all about being angry with Johnny and me, and we saw him and Marie fairly often. One day we were coming out of a casino after a show, and Leonard began to follow people around. He was following some ladies, and when they went into the ladies' rest room, Leonard went right in with them. It caused quite a stir. He and Marie were staying at a motel, and when Leonard forgot which room was his, he just walked down the hall knocking on every single door to see which one was his. People thought he was some kind of pervert or something. Nobody expects to see someone in his forties with Alzheimer's disease. People expect that very old people are the only ones who have it. Ninety percent of the public doesn't know anything about Alzheimer's disease anyway. They just see this guy acting strange, and it's scary.

Marie told about a time when it was trash day, and Leonard went down the entire block, gathering up all the trash containers from all the neighbors and lining them up in front of their house. When a man who looks fairly young and healthy does these crazy things, people don't know what to think.

After Leonard married Marie, his condition disintegrated quite rapidly. He was unruly and belligerent one day, and then passive and clinging the next. Marie was bitter at us for not telling her that he might have Alzheimer's disease. I can understand how she feels, but Johnny and I still wonder if she would have listened if we had said anything.

Marie took good care of Leonard. She had a board and care home for the elderly and knew how to take care of people. After a time, Leonard became so difficult that it was finally too much for Marie, and she had to find a facility that would take him.

One night shortly after midnight, Leonard had started to move all the furniture outside. It was pouring down rain. When Marie tried to stop him, he turned on her and tried to choke her. She pulled free and hurriedly called 911. When the police arrived, Leonard calmed down immediately. The officer took Leonard by the hand and walked him to the police car. Leonard offered no resistance. Maybe Leonard responded to the uniform as a symbol of authority. Maybe he had forgotten what he was doing. He certainly had forgotten that he was angry with his wife. In any case, Leonard never returned home.

From the crisis center where he was taken by the police, Marie placed him in a nursing home. She visited him regularly, and I visited as often as I could.

I'll never forget the first time I visited Leonard in a convalescent home. Dealing with one individual at a time was difficult enough. To go into a nursing home and see about a hundred-sixty demented people in one place was shocking and depressing. It just about took my breath away. Some were walking around without their clothes. Others were half dressed. One woman took off her panties and came up to me and handed them to me. I didn't know what to do. Some patients were mumbling to themselves. Others were sitting in a dazed stupor. It was overwhelming. It was all I could do to keep from crying.

On top of the shock of seeing all these people, the place was filthy. The carpet was spotted and stained and reeked of urine. If I live to be a hundred, I'll never forget that smell. I could hardly breathe. To this day, when I go into a nursing home that has that smell, that first visit to see Leonard comes back to me, and I become so depressed. To see my brother in this place broke my heart, but there was nothing else to do. Nobody in the family had money for private care, and it had become impossible for him to be cared for at home.

It was about one hundred ten degrees. Sacramento gets very hot in the summer. I found Leonard sitting in a wheel chair dressed in a wool robe. I was angry. Alzheimer's patients are helpless when it comes to taking care of themselves. There was no way Leonard could change his uncomfortable clothing, or even explain that he wanted a change or that he was miserable. I found an aide, and asked her how she would like to be sitting out in the heat in a wool robe. She wheeled Leonard in and changed him into something cooler and more comfortable. But he never should have been in that wool robe in the first place. I was beside myself.

One day Tommy Lou and I were visiting, and we took Leonard for a walk around the grounds. He kept repeating in a plaintive voice, "I wanta go home. I wanta go home. Take me home." It is so common for Alzheimer's patients to say they want to go home. They all want to go home, but nevertheless, it broke our hearts. We felt so guilty, but we couldn't take him home. I know now that Leonard really wanted to go home to Kansas City, and there was no way he could do that. Still, I was so sad to hear him beg to go home. Today, I would tell him, "Okay, we'll go home in a little while." Then I would ask one of the staff for a cookie or something to give him. At least he would have been happy for a little while.

Marie told how he would get down on his hands and knees and try to dig under the fence. He kept telling her again and again, "I wanta go home." He didn't do that when we were there. Thank God. I don't know what I would have done if I'd seen him do that. It was hard enough just having him in that home. He did stoop down and take a handful of leaves and start to eat them. To see our own brother in such a state that he couldn't tell what was food and what wasn't was horrible. When we left, Tommy Lou and I stood outside of the nursing home and clung to each other and sobbed.

About five years later, I was asked to speak to the staff and a support group at that same place. I had not been back since Leonard had left there. When I drove up, I realized which place this was, and I just sat in the car and repeated over and over to Johnny, "I can't go in. I just can't. The place is terrible. I can't stand it, going in here again. It's so depressing. I can't bear it. Johnny, please, I can't go in." I was crying like a baby by then. The people inside were waiting for me.

As usual, Johnny was calm and comforting. He talked and talked to me, reassuring me.

"The reason we're back here, Bea, is because they have made a lot of changes. It is a different place now. It is designed just for Alzheimer's patients now. They want us to see the changes. They want us to know how it is now so that we can tell other people about it. If we don't go in, Bea, and see the changes they've made, we can't recommend it. People need to know about places that are caring and well run. If we don't know which ones they are, we can't help people. We must go in, Bea. You'll be okay once you go inside. It is not the same as it was. We need to see that for ourselves."

He was right. Once I got inside, I was all right. The place was freshly painted and clean. The rug was gone. The smell was gone. The patients were clean. They were not medicated to the point where they were sitting around in a drugged stupor. They seemed more content. The staff were obviously working hard to provide good care. They were learning. They were sincerely trying. These people obviously cared about their patients. A woman named Cynda Rennie was the new activities coordinator. She and I became good friends. Cynda told me later that, had she known my brother had been there, she never would have asked me to come without finding out how I might feel about being there. We need more people like Cynda.

I remembered that, when Leonard had been there, the place had been horrible. The comfort I felt in seeing the changes that had taken place was heart warming. To know that there are places like this for Alzheimer's patients was reassuring. Things were getting better.

When Leonard was no longer ambulatory, he was moved to another facility, which was as bad as the first place. There he was confined to his bed. Whenever Johnny and I were in Sacramento, which was at least once a month for the support group meetings, I would visit my brother. We were running late one day, so Johnny double parked and stayed in the car with the engine idling while I dashed in for a brief visit.

I went into Leonard's room, and there he was, naked, wet, and soiled. The stench was awful. He had no way to pull up the sheet to cover himself. He was unable to call for help. I had no idea how long he had been lying there. It was late afternoon when I arrived. He could have been lying there like that all day. That's the heart breaking thing about Alzheimer's disease. The loss of dignity. The helplessness. Anybody can do anything they want to those victims, and there's absolutely nothing they can do. If the family doesn't fight for their care, who will? Nursing homes are improving, but there is still a lot of bad care out there.

I ran out to the car and told Johnny that I had to do something about Leonard. He parked and came in. I found several nurses or aides at the nurses station and told them about my brother. One of them went immediately and took care of him. I was relieved to see that they bathed him and dressed him, but what if I hadn't come? I couldn't be there every day to see that they took good care of him. The whole thing made me sad, guilty, and depressed. I would be upset whenever I thought about Leonard's situation.

If you have a loved one in a home, visit often. I think they will get better care that way. When the staff knows you are going to come in, and if you don't like something, you're going to say something, I believe a person gets better care. Now there are more and more places that give good care no matter whether an individual has any visitors or not, but it still is good to visit as often as you can.

Leonard died almost a year after he was bedridden. When he died, Marie offered his body to research, and felt that maybe some good could come out of this tragedy if medical scientists could study Leonard's brain. She called all the family and explained, suggesting that each arrange a memorial service as they saw fit. Evelyn and Leonard's children are still quite bitter because they didn't have Leonard's body for burial. They feel that their daddy just was gone, and they didn't have a chance to mourn. Even though his children don't understand, they may feel differently when they realize that their father's suffering wasn't in vain, and that others may have been helped by Marie's decision.

Dr. William Ellis of the University of California Davis Medical Center recently told us that he continues to receive requests from researchers all over the country for samples of Leonard's brain tissue. The fact that Leonard had familial Alzheimer's makes this tissue especially important. Dr. Ellis feels that Leonard continues to contribute significantly in the search for a cure. Hopefully, there are children growing up today who will be saved from having to suffer as Leonard had suffered. Maybe his own grandchildren.

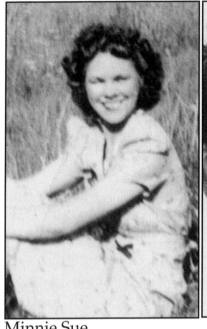

Minnie Sue

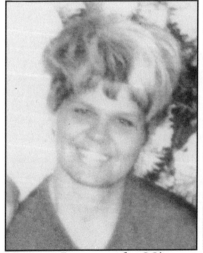

Johnny & Bea, age 40

Norma Jean, early 30's

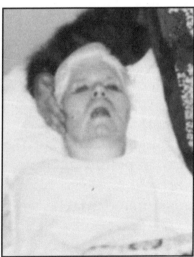

Norma Jean

CHAPTER THIRTEEN

Norma Jean

Norma Jean, like her sisters Tommy Lou and Mary, was a beauty. She was tiny, just over five feet tall and slender. When she smiled, her face lit up and her eyes sparkled. She laughed easily and often. She was undemanding, sweet, and easy going. I always remember Norma as being an easy person to be around.

Soon after Mama died, Norma Jean took off for Hollywood to visit Tommy Lou and Mary. Once there, she took a job at Paramount Studios working as a clerk in the payroll department. Later she worked as a secretary for Vasserette, a bra manufacturer popular in the forties and fifties. Her shapely body was not lost on company bosses, and attending various Hollywood functions as a model and company representative, sort of a goodwill ambassador, of the Vasserette Company was added to her line of duties. It was a fantastic job, and Norma Jean loved it. Being paid to be social and meet all kinds of people was the kind of job most single girls would die for. It was at one of these receptions that she met Ed, the man she would marry, and she never returned to Kansas City.

Ed was educated and ambitious. He had dreams of starting a business, and there was little doubt that he would be successful. He was also attracted to this petite, unspoiled, beauty whose sparkle and laughter pleased him. Norma Jean idolized Ed. For Norma, Ed was a dream-come-true. Although Ed was quite shy, Norma Jean saw him as worldly and sophisticated.

Both Norma Jean and Ed came from poor families. Ed grew up in Hanover, New Hampshire. Most of his friends' dads and a few of their moms worked at Dartmouth College. They were professors or heads of departments, researchers or secretaries. Ed's dad worked at Dartmouth, too. He drove the trash truck. His family lived at the end of the road east of town. Although Ed was active and successful in sports, captain of the basketball team, and accepted by his classmates, he was keenly aware of their differences, not only in affluence, but in status. Ed was also bound and determined to make a different life for himself. After a stint in the military, and testing in the nineties on the Veteran's college entrance exam, he enrolled at the University of New Hampshire. He was the first one in his family, not only to finish high school, but to attend college.

At the end of his junior year, Ed returned to Hanover, unable to finish his senior year because of financial difficulties. Soon, a call came telling Ed to go talk to the president of the local Rotary club. They had money to lend him for school. Another call came from the local bank. Another from a local business. Money to cover the costs of his final year was available. He returned for his senior year and graduated with a degree in forestry.

High school friends had parents in the right places and in the right organizations. High school friends had come through for the kid who lived at the end of the road east of town without his ever asking. Ed would never have asked, but he appreciated the help when it came. After graduating, he worked in Alaska for a year. His first job was to pay back those who had lent him money and made it possible for him to finish school.

In 1953, after working in the Northwest and in Washington DC, he found his way to Southern California and decided to make his home in the land of sunshine and orange trees. Three years later, he met Norma Jean King.

In Norma, he found someone from a similar background, someone who understood what it was like to grow up poor. They could learn together, grow together. They had come from the same place. They could climb the same mountains. They could be partners in business as well as marriage and, together, they could change their lives. Besides, Ed was in his early thirties and eager to settle down. It was time. He wanted his share of the American dream. He wanted a family, a wife and kids, and here was this beautiful woman pressuring him to do just that. After dating for almost two years, Ed and Norma married on February 1, 1958. Norma Jean was twenty-eight years old.

Their early years of marriage were good years. They had a budget and a plan. First they would save to have a nest egg. Then they would begin making investments. Buying an apartment house was their first step. The second step was to start a business. Once established, they bought their first home. With these things accomplished, they would begin their family. Both were eager to have children.

Their two sons arrived sixteen months apart. Ed and Norma Jean were thrilled. Ed worked hard to build his business. Norma took care of the household and the boys. Ed was determined to improve himself and his lot, and he looked to his wife to be his partner. He wanted her help in the daily operation of the business and in the entertaining of successful clients. Norma Jean, on the other hand, had failed to graduate from high school and had neither the ambition nor the desire to continue her education or learn more sophisticated ways. She lacked the social skills Ed sought and needed in a wife.

He wanted to share the responsibilities as well as the rewards. She just wanted to be married to Ed. She was content. Striving for what Ed saw as "the good life" required hard work. Norma didn't understand how much work was involved. She was ill prepared to be a full partner in their struggle to build that life her husband sought. As far as Norma was concerned, they already had the good life.

In the beginning, Ed saw only her beauty, her laughter, and her delightful smile. He found her innocence refreshing. One evening, when picking up the tab for dinner, Ed was amused to find that Norma Jean had never seen a one-hundred-dollar bill before. In time, he became less amused and more critical of her naiveté. Norma "didn't have any gumption." To him, she appeared to have no interest in what he was working so hard to accomplish, no drive to achieve, and she didn't seem to care whether he succeeded or not.

Norma Jean did care in her way. She idolized her husband. It was just that she didn't care in the way Ed needed for her to care. In a very few years, Ed saw mostly her shortcomings, but by that time, she was the mother of their two sons. Their first boy was born on Norma Jean's thirtieth birthday.

Ed was devoted to his sons, and knowing the value of education, saw to it that they attended the best schools. From primary grades through college, they had the best education money could buy. Both boys would graduate from leading universities.

While the boys were still in grade school, Norma Jean's temperament seemed to be changing. She became distracted and was easily upset. We look back now and wonder just when the illness began. Was she getting sick or was she dissatisfied with her life? What caused the outbreaks of anger? Was she being irrational or was she just tired? No one really knew. We just knew the changes were there. With the onset of her illness, her social ineptness would be exaggerated.

I believe now that Norma Jean knew before anyone else knew that something was wrong with her.
When she lashed out at Ed, she could feel him pull
away from her. When he did, in her insecurity, she
would react by clinging to him more tightly. Her moods
were unpredictable. Her responses irrational. Her behavior unreliable. All was not well with Ed and Norma.

Johnny and I knew that Ed was having problems with Norma, and we didn't want to admit that
we suspected her problems might be early signs of
Alzheimer's disease. We know now that we should
have talked to Ed. We should have, but we didn't.
Maybe we could have lessened his trauma by explaining the cause of his wife's craziness and letting him
know what to expect in the future. But I wasn't ready
to admit that Norma Jean might be sick.

Johnny and I think now that Ed was waiting for
us to say that something was wrong with Norma Jean,
but we wouldn't. We didn't want to believe that
Alzheimer's disease was striking our family again. We
were in denial. But deep down in our souls, we knew
it. We wondered briefly if Ed would have listened to
us if we had talked to him. But Ed is an intelligent man,
open to learning, and deep down, we knew he would
have listened. We just didn't say anything, and we
should have.

When the wife of a couple who were friends of
Norma Jean and Ed developed multiple sclerosis, the
husband left. He just up and took off, and nobody ever

heard from him again. Norma was extremely distraught when the husband, Joe, abandoned his sick wife. The wife died a few years later. It was soon after Joe left, one evening when Ed and Norma Jean were at a restaurant having dinner, that she looked at Ed across the table, and, very simply and directly, said, "I have the disease."

Ed watched his frightened wife as she sat still and silent. "You're not married to Joe, Norma. You're married to Ed," he said. "I will never leave you, Norma."

That painful but reassuring encounter led to one of the closest periods of their marriage. But Alzheimer's disease is relentless. Good times are never allowed to last. The disease is always the winner. As Norma Jean's personality deteriorated, closeness gave way to dissension.

Ed knew what was happening to his wife and began his own education on Alzheimer's disease. He faced the challenge of supporting and caring for two sons and a disabled wife. His commitment to providing good care was strong. She was his responsibility, and he accepted that responsibility. So began his task of learning how to care for a victim of Alzheimer's disease. He attended seminars. He read everything he could find.

I still wasn't ready to face the truth. If you include our mama, four of our family had already fallen prey. When would it stop? If Norma Jean was number five, who would be number six? Or number seven?

When would it end? No. There was no way in the world I could admit that Norma Jean was in the early stages of Alzheimer's disease.

While I am denying that my sister is ill, Norma Jean is stopping at the supermarket while her boys are waiting in the car. Sometimes they would be kept waiting for almost an hour as she struggled to remember where to find a quart of milk or tried to make a decision on what brand of cereal to purchase. When she came out of the market, she would invariably have difficulty finding the car.

Ed brought Norma Jean to stay with us while he went on a scouting trip with the boys. She felt abandoned and rejected and wanted to know why she couldn't join her family. She couldn't, of course, because the trip was for boys and their fathers, not their mothers. There weren't any women going, but Norma Jean couldn't accept that. She fussed and fumed. Then she wanted to return to Los Angeles to take care of the business. She wanted us to drive her there immediately. Norma Jean was full of unreasonable demands. We were full of unreasonable responses. Norma Jean wouldn't listen. We kept trying to figure out some way to get her home safely. None of our suggestions were acceptable.

Kim, home from college, tapped my shoulder and pointed to her aunt who was sitting in the corner chair sobbing. I asked Norma Jean what was the matter, and she just sobbed louder. Then she started having one screaming fit.

"You don't want me here!" she shouted at me. "No one wants me! Ed doesn't want me! Nobody! Nobody wants me!" By now, she was hysterical. We were hurt because all I was trying to do was to help her.

If we had known then what we know now, we wouldn't have tried to solve her problem. We would just have listened, and then talked softly to her and diverted her attention to something else. We would have offered her cookies or ice cream or told her how pretty her hair looked. We would have done something to take her mind off her problem, and she would soon have forgotten all about it. But no. We did the worst possible thing. We accepted her accusations and tried to argue with her. Our actions only made things worse. We know now that the thing to do is to distract someone who has Alzheimer's disease. Diversion is the best defense against the irrationality of the disease.

But we didn't do that. Instead, I called Tommy Lou to come with me. Until Tommy Lou arrived, Norma Jean sat and played solitaire. She scarcely said a word. Later, she would forget how to play, but I was glad at the time that she still remembered. As I look back on that incident, I doubt if she played the game with any accuracy. I am sure that black sixes weren't going on red sevens, but that didn't matter. Playing solitaire kept her busy for hours.

Tommy Lou and I drove our sister to Bishop to meet someone who would drive her home to Los Angeles. When we started our drive back home, we could no longer deny the truth. Her sons were in high school, and by now, there was no question in their minds or anyone else's that their mother was ill. It was time that I admitted the truth. Norma Jean was victim number five.

For years, she had golfed every Wednesday with three of her women friends. Suddenly the other women stopped playing, evidently because they had had enough of Norma Jean's erratic behavior. Ed asked them about it, and although he didn't get a direct answer, he knew.

The weird stuff continued. She saved cereal boxes and had a fit if anyone wanted to throw any of them out. The back and sides of the garage were stacked to the ceiling with cereal boxes.

Norma Jean talked with great animation about her daughters. She went on and on, in great detail, giving them names and personalities. Norma Jean didn't have any daughters.

Ed continued his own education. He and Norma Jean became involved in research at the University of California at Los Angeles Medical School. He volunteered to become a control subject in their research project, so when they tested Norma, they also tested Ed. He did everything possible to help. He read. He went to lectures. He attended support groups, and he translated all he learned into the best possible care for his wife.

Ed was a frequent volunteer in the boys' scouting activities. The more he participated in his boys' lives, the more Norma Jean clung to him for attention. She felt abandoned and insecure. The more she clung, the more difficult she became.

One time while Norma Jean could still be at home by herself during the day, Johnny and I stopped to visit them. Norma wanted to take us to lunch. The restaurant was nearby, so we decided to walk. Norma Jean could still walk by herself every day and not become lost. She would take us to the restaurant which was a short block away.

We were concerned when she started off in the opposite direction, but since she walked every day, we followed. She took us about eight blocks out of our way before reaching the restaurant. That was her normal route, and she was unable to change it and maintain her orientation.

We ate lunch and chatted. More accurately, Johnny and I chatted and Norma Jean said very little. Her ability to speak was diminishing, so she couldn't really carry on a conversation. When the bill arrived, she offered to pay with a bunch of pennies. It looked to me that she had about fifty, obviously, not enough to buy lunch for three people. She opened her coin purse and dumped the stack of pennies on a napkin. It was clear that Norma Jean was totally "out of touch." Johnny paid the bill, we thanked Norma Jean for taking us to lunch, and the three of us walked back to Norma's and Ed's house.

Soon after that day, Norma Jean was taking her routine walk when she became disoriented and lost.

She did know enough to go into a store and phone her husband. She remembered his phone number at work, and they made the call for her. Ed came immediately and took his wife home. After that, he bought her an ID bracelet with a stone in it. A rhinestone, but a stone nevertheless. It also had her name, address, home phone, and Ed's phone number at work. Norma Jean loved that bracelet and would tell everybody, "Look what Ed gave me. Isn't it beautiful? It's got a diamond." She wouldn't take it off, which was precisely what Ed wanted.

That's where we got the idea for ID bracelets. From Ed. Make the bracelet like a piece of jewelry and make a fancy gift of it. Fancy and special. Never put any identification about illness. Patient's become angry and resentful and will refuse to wear something that labels them as "being sick." Johnny and I always tell people to give the bracelet as a gift. That way, there is a better chance that the person who has Alzheimer's disease will treasure it and wear it.

Not too long after getting lost, Norma Jean became more and more afraid to walk alone. She continued to deteriorate. From time to time, Tommy Lou would come down from Vallejo to help care for her. Tommy would also take Norma Jean back to Vallejo, sometimes for a month or more at a time. For years, Ed took Norma Jean to work with him when she could no longer be left home alone and couldn't travel to visit Tommy Lou. Finally, Norma Jean was not able to come into the office, and Ed hired someone to take care of her at home. It was not until near the end of her life, when Norma Jean was completely helpless, that she was placed in a nursing home. By then she needed to be where skilled professionals had the resources and proper equipment to provide the care she required.

Norma Jean lived longer than any of the others in our family who had Alzheimer's disease. Johnny and I always said that it was because she had such good care. She died on May 26, 1992. It has always seemed ironic to me that she gave birth to her younger son on her thirty-second birthday, and she died on her older son's thirtieth birthday.

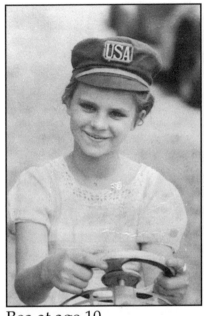

Bea at age 10

Bea & Johnny

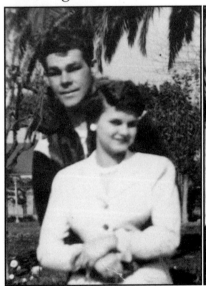

Bea & brother Leonard

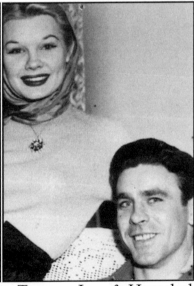

Tommy Lou & Herschel

CHAPTER FOURTEEN

The Alzheimer's Aid Society Today

From our floundering and humble beginnings, The Alzheimer's Aid Society has continued to grow. I think back to our second support group meeting held on May 8, 1981, where Dr. Bob Cook-Deegan and Dr. Pierre Dreyfus were our speakers, and remember being thrilled and excited to have such important and knowledgeable people as speakers at our new organization. Both of them continue to be leaders in research on Alzheimer's disease. Both are dedicated men who took time from their busy schedules to speak to a fledgling group, a group that was not yet really organized. They set a very high standard for us, and we have continued to seek out outstanding people in the fields of Alzheimer's research, care, and caregiver support.

Ramona Denney, who later became secretary of our organization, arranged for us to hold the meeting at the church where her brother was pastor. She brought us an expando file for our papers and a recipe-like box to hold three-by-five cards for organizing names and addresses. We were starting off at ground zero. I smile when I remember this first step in putting together a mailing list. Today, our list is constantly being cleaned and updated, with names being removed as patients and caregivers pass on, and new names added as calls come in for help and people join our support groups. The latest count is over twelve thousand names. We have had over fifteen thousand names. The list is on computer and is bar coded. I feel very high tech!

When we began, our offices were the dining room in our home. Today, we have offices in Lodi and Sacramento. When we were overflowing into the living room, the bedrooms and kitchen, Johnny asked the Department of Aging at the state where he might find donated office space. Within an hour, he received a call from Shirley Kleim. She put us in touch with William Holz, who had dedicated his time, his money, and his heart and soul to helping the elderly. He had built the Loel Community Senior Center and was eager to provide us with office space. This space would be rent free, but we would pay our share of utilities. That sounded more than fair to us. Our prayers had been answered.

Shirley was a blessing beyond description to us and to our struggling organization. She is one of the most upbeat people I have ever met. Her goodness and love for people radiate. Her laughter is always spontaneous. I look back and wonder if we would have made it without her. She has done and continues to do so much for us.

We have been in the Loel Center now since 1984. Today, our office is wall-to-wall desks and files, copier, fax, and phones, bulletin boards, books, videos, and printed information, but we're happy here and don't plan to move. I can walk to the post office, the printer, the type setter, our legal advisor, and to the jeweler who engraves our ID bracelets. Lodi is a friendly town, and the convenient location of our office is a blessing.

Shirley introduced us to the world of volunteers, a gold mine of eager hearts and hands ready to help. Today, these wonderful people are essential in keeping the organization going.

The Sacramento office is open five days a week and staffed entirely by volunteers. When one person can't make it to the office, someone else covers. If they're stranded and can't get anybody, we cover the office. The same thing happens when a facilitator can't make it to a support group meeting. If at all possible, Johnny and I will cover for them.

The Lodi office is where we do the bulk of the "nuts-and-bolts" work. The newsletter is printed and sent out from Lodi, as is the printed information we provide to support groups. We have a library of videos, tapes, and books here, as well as in the Sacramento office. Generous, helpful volunteers make it all possible.

The volunteers are marvelous people. We couldn't get along without them. They facilitate support groups, help with sending out all of the mailings, keeping the mailing lists updated on the computer, organizing workshops, answering phones, and listening when someone needs to talk. The Alzheimer's Aid Society averages about seven hundred hours a month of volunteer time. That is the same as having over four full-time employees. By the time an organization pays salaries and payroll taxes, let alone benefits, those volunteers would cost about $85,000 a year. Of course, we couldn't afford that and still provide services at little or no cost.

Recognizing people once a year doesn't begin to show how much we appreciate all the help these people give, but once a year, we have a volunteer appreciation day. Believe me, we appreciate them every day!

In Sacramento, lunch is provided by a different nursing home each year. Johnny does all the cooking for the volunteer dinners in Lodi. It's quite an occasion.

As the Alzheimer's Aid Society continues to grow, we know the day will come when we'll have to hire a full-time person to help run things. It's getting to be more than the two of us, even with so many volunteers, can handle.

We receive an average of over fifteen hundred phone calls a month. When the office closes, we transfer the calls to our home. That way, the phone is answered twenty-four hours a day. When a person is desperate for help, it is important that there is someone available to respond.

Over 125,000 pieces of literature a year, including our newsletter, are sent out from our office. We have an extensive library of videos and tapes available on a loan basis to support groups and individuals. Our small reference library offers books on the same basis. We contribute financially to Alzheimer's research being carried on at Universities of California at Davis, Berkeley, and San Diego. We provide supplies, such as diapers, to those in need who cannot afford to purchase them, as well as financial assistance for respite care in needy situations.

For the last six years, Johnny has spoken to from three to seven groups a week, sometimes giving as many as four presentations in one day. He speaks to service clubs, to nursing home staffs, the nursing students at the Delta College and at National University in Sacramento, to professional organizations, owners of board and care facilities, church groups, and retirement organizations.

Johnny organizes trips to research laboratories for members and facilitators from the support groups. For example, on one trip we visited University of California at Berkeley and the Veteran's Hospital in Palo Alto. We had contacted them ahead of time, of course, and they had speakers ready for us. The doctors were wonderful. They spoke to our group and updated us on the research being done. We were given a tour of their laboratories. They even served us lunch. It is so very encouraging for those who live with this disease to see the efforts being made toward finding a cure.

Johnny and I meet with an average of ten families a month and make home visits between two and three times a week. Most of our calls for help, about seventy percent, are from in-laws, close friends of the caregiver, or someone else not in the immediate family. It is often easier to see strange patterns of behavior when you're not with a person everyday. Often immediate family members are in denial. Sometimes a person has Alzheimer's disease for three to five years before the family acknowledges that something is definitely wrong. It is difficult to face the possibility that someone dear to you could be a victim of this terrifying disease.

Recently we were speaking with a man who, after years of denial, had finally faced the painful fact that his wife had Alzheimer's disease. They were flying from Sacramento to Tokyo, at thirty-two thousand feet in the air, when his wife got out of her seat, turned to her husband, and said, "I'm going outside for a smoke. "His period of denial ended abruptly.

When Johnny and I meet with families, we ask that all family members attend if possible. If everyone understands what is happening to Mom or Dad or Aunt Tillie or Uncle Bill or Grandma or Grandpa, and what the immediate caregiver is going through, other family members are usually more supportive. It is terribly hard on a caregiver to do all the work of caring for the one who has Alzheimer's disease and then have other members of the family criticize them. It's hard to believe, but it happens far more often than we like to admit. Some member of the family will blame the caregiver for the illness and criticize the caregiver's actions. "Aunt Tillie is enough to drive any one crazy. Poor Uncle Bill. Nothing's wrong with him if she'd just get off his back and quit nagging at him." The one who usually deserves your love and consideration is Aunt Tillie.

Johnny and I explain what they can expect will happen as the illness progresses, and some of the things that they can do that might help them cope with the loved one needing care and with their own discouragement. Caregivers need to know they are not alone in their stress and suffering, their guilt and frustration. Caregivers need to learn to take care of themselves as they face this grueling task of being a caregiver.

We provide printed information and recommend books to read, tell families about local support groups, when they meet, and where. We offer the use of videos and tapes and books. And we explain that we are there for them when they need us.

We also listen. Facing Alzheimer's disease is a dreadful experience, and it is important to have understanding and knowledgeable people to talk to. Besides, once people have been through this terrible experience, they have a lot of compassion for others who are facing the same thing. Until a person has been there, it's difficult to know what it is like.

We explain that Alzheimer's patients are wanderers and frequently become lost. We have started an

Elder Identification program with nineteen senior centers cooperating with us. Three pictures no larger than 3″ x 3″ along with the physical description of the victim of the disease and the address and phone number of the caregiver are kept on file at the local police department, the Alzheimer's Aid Society, and a designated senior center in the local area. Some families also provide their Alzheimer's victims with ID bracelets, which is an added help in bringing a lost person home. By working with police and local senior centers, search time for a lost loved one is greatly reduced. Response to this program has been very positive.

Once a year, we offer one major workshop at American River College in Sacramento, and three to four mini-workshops in various locations throughout the area. We have been filled to capacity for the last two, with over four hundred people attending. It looks as though we will have to move to larger facilities soon.

Leading physicians, social workers, gerontologists, medical researchers, registered nurses, and other knowledgeable individuals involved in working with Alzheimer's patients are presenters. Topics we cover each time include: Update on Research usually presented by a leading neurologist, Elder Law presented by an attorney who specializes in Elder Law, Dealing with Grief and Guilt presented by social workers or psychologists, Care of the Alzheimer's Victim is presented by an individual with extensive experience in successful care of Alzheimer's patients. Other topics may include <u>Drug Information</u>, <u>Looking for a Nursing Home</u>, <u>Incontinence Care Information</u>, <u>Handling Stress</u>, <u>Sexuality and the Alzheimer's Patient</u>, <u>Hospice Care</u>, <u>Legislation</u>, <u>Activities for the Alzheimer's Patient</u>. The workshops offer a variety of speakers and topics with helpful information.

The Alzheimer's Aid Society has remained independent. We considered joining the national organization, but for us, being independent has allowed us to do what we felt was most important in our community. If people want to, they can organize themselves and make a difference. They can reach out and help others. They can meet the needs of their local community. By being independent, we don't have to follow anyone else's guidelines. For example, we don't charge for membership in the organization. We're not saying that charging for membership is wrong, it is just that we didn't want to go in that direction. We do raise money, but on a donation basis. When we are asked to speak on television or serve on a panel, we are free to do so. We don't need permission from a parent organization. On the other hand, some groups find belonging to a larger organization very helpful. The need is great, and there's room for all of us.

Johnny and I would like to see the independent support group organizations form a loosely structured network. Independent Alzheimer's groups from all over the country could share ideas which could help all of us serve caregivers and victims of Alzheimer's disease more effectively. We have talked with other groups who operate independently and have found that they are very interested. As soon as John and I can slow down long enough to catch our breath, we want to help form a network for exchanging ideas and exploring new ways for finding more resources.

Along the way, we have met many people who are life's treasures. As with any treasures, they make our lives infinitely richer. They are people we never would have met had we not set out on this course to help victims of Alzheimer's disease. They are, to us, God's blessings. We have mentioned several. This book would not be complete without also mentioning Pat Warner. She owns and directs the Curry Manor in Roseburg, Oregon. Curry Manor is an inspiration to caregivers everywhere where creative solutions are everyday events. Pat's enthusiasm and knowledge, her ideas and her love for people have inspired many, including Johnny and me. She has spoken to groups around the country, including our workshops. Although the ideas we offer that might be helpful to caregivers and family members have come from multiple sources, many have originated with Pat Warner.

Johnny and I keep busy and our work is rewarding. It is important that we provide support for the caregiver, but it is also important that we continue to educate people about Alzheimer's disease. Movies about Alzheimer's disease sometimes dramatize the illness. One made a romantic love story that didn't begin to show the ugly reality of Alzheimer's disease. Food drooling out the mouth. The vacant stare. The rages. The meaningless mumbling that has replaced the ability to talk. The loss of control of bodily functions. The demanding, clinging, whining behavior. Aggression and violence. The disintegration of a personality. Alzheimer's disease is ugly.

It is important that the general population understand. It is not uncommon for a caregiver to say nothing about a mother or father or spouse who has Alzheimer's disease. They often keep silent about their plight. They are afraid to speak out. They are embarrassed to have their loved ones lose their minds.

For years, Alzheimer's disease has been considered an illness for old people. An attitude exists that says, "What's the point of spending so much money since their lives are almost over anyway? What's the use? They're old anyway." That attitude is slowly changing as people learn more about the disease. That is why the story must be told. It must be told again and again until enough people know and demand that more be done to help caregivers and victims.

We can learn a great deal from victims of AIDS. Where Alzheimer's patients have lost the ability to fight for their cause, AIDS patients are young. Their minds are intact. They have made their cause known. They have demanded that dollars be spent to find a cure. In April of 1986, it was reported in the *Sacramento Bee* that in California, AIDS, which affected approximately 4,000 persons, was allocated $7.2 million dollars in the state budget for research and care. Alzheimer's disease, which affected approximately 250,000 people, received $250,000. That ratio has changed. We are grateful to learn the importance of education and public awareness that those who are working to find a cure for AIDS have taught us. That education leads to compassion and understanding.

It is important that we continue to tell the horror stories of Alzheimer's disease so that people will know. So that caregivers will receive help. So that research dollars will be committed. So that a cure and even prevention will be found. The public must know the truth about Alzheimer's disease.

CHAPTER FIFTEEN

Our Lives Today

Today, Johnny and I live in Lodi, California, just two miles from the offices donated to us in the Loel Community Center. We settled here in 1983 when Johnny was transferred to a supermarket in Lodi. I love it here. Lodi may not be as beautiful as Lake Tahoe, but it never snows, and the roads are never icy. It is hot in the summer, but that suits me just fine. Lodi is a friendly town, and we're happy to live here. Our kids are grown, but three out of four live nearby. Jack is in Washington DC, where he is a lobbyist for higher education. We get back there to see him as often as we can. Kim, Wendy, and John Jr., live in the area, and we see them often. Kim finished her master's degree and works as a sales representative for a large pharmaceutical company. John Jr. owns his own business. Wendy is caring full time for an elderly woman who has Alzheimer's disease. The grandchildren count is at six, and we work hard to adore and spoil them.

Early every morning, five-o'clock-in-the-morn-
ing early, Johnny and I walk for forty-five minutes, and
again each evening, we do the same. We had both put
on too many extra pounds, and when Johnny had a
heart attack, we decided it was time to do something
about it.

We always walk hand-in-hand. Recently, we
passed someone who said we looked so happy, holding hands and all, and they wondered if we were new-
lyweds. I had to laugh. I explained that I hold Johnny's
hand so he won't run off and leave me, and he holds
my hand so I won't go back and sit on the couch and
watch television. It is a good system.

In 1993, Johnny and I celebrated our fortieth
wedding anniversary. Johnny's sister had called to say
that she and her husband Sam were coming from Kansas City to Tahoe to celebrate Sam's birthday, and they
asked us to join them. Our anniversary and his birthday are on the same day, and she thought it would be
fun to celebrate together.

Pauline and Sam came first to our place in Lodi.
She explained that we all had to be in Tahoe at a certain time for Sam's birthday dinner party. If we arrived
any earlier, he might start gambling, and it would be
hard to get him away from the gambling tables for the
party. That all seemed a little strange, but I didn't argue.

I had called the kids to see if any of them would
join us. They all had other plans. I was so hurt. You've

probably figured out by now that I get hurt rather easily. The night before we left, I sat with my sister-and brother-in-law and moaned and groaned and bad mouthed my kids something terrible. I didn't want to go to Tahoe anyway, but now I felt bound to go. It was all very complicated.

We arrived at the designated time. I wasn't in a celebrating mood and was annoyed with myself that I had agreed to go. When Johnny and I entered the room where we were to attend this birthday party for Sam, I couldn't believe my eyes. There were over one hundred people in the room. My kids and their spouses and our grand kids, my sisters, Mary, Tommy Lou, and Anna June, Sonny and his family, our friends from Kansas City and from Denver, as well as from Tahoe and Lodi. There were volunteers and support group facilitators. There were nieces and nephews galore and their kids. There were Ed, Norma Jean's husband, and his boys, Evelyn, Leonard's first wife, and Anna Sue, Minnie Sue's daughter from Kansas City. Johnny's sisters, Pauline and Teresa Ann, came and his nephew Brian and his son were there from Colorado. It was quite a crowd.

I was speechless. I wondered if Johnny had known anything about this and didn't tell me, but he hadn't known anything either and was as surprised as I was. The hall was decorated with streamers and balloons. It was very festive. There was live music. Sonny recorded the entire thing on video tape.

For a family that isn't supposed to be very close, they sure turned out for our anniversary party. I was so touched. I guess we have a pretty close family after all. After walking around the room hugging everybody, we took our seats at the head table.

John Jr. was the first to speak. First he told about all the phone calls they had made, and had they ever made phone calls! Kim kept calling him, and John Jr. would tell her, "I've got it covered. I've got it covered!" Everyone was laughing, and the next thing I knew, we were all wiping tears from our eyes. John Jr. paid tribute to us and then went on to say that he always wanted a marriage like his mom and dad have, so he searched for the perfect wife and found Arlene so that he could have the same kind of relationship Johnny and I have. He wanted to have the same relationship with his kids that we have with our kids. He wanted to be the kind of dad Johnny was, and he wanted Arlene to be the kind of mom I was. He said, "My parents have done everything to help us," and then he started to choke up. Jack was next to me. He reached over and picked up a napkin from the table and wiped his eyes.

John Jr. continued. "They shared their love in every way. I tell my friends that my dad went to every ball game I ever played, and they say, 'What d'ya mean, every game?' They couldn't believe it.

"My mom went to two games. The first one she went to, I broke my leg, and at the second one, I left in an ambulance. That was her last game. She couldn't stand to see me get hurt. That second time, she decided she'd better quit coming before I got myself killed."

Kim read notes people had written telling things they remember about us. Tommy Lou remembered coming home from Hollywood and always kissing me on the bridge of my nose, and everyone in the neighborhood knew Tommy Lou was home because of the lipstick on my nose. I wept when Kim read Anna June's letter recalling how I had given her my wedding dress so she could cut it up and make a dress for her wedding to Leon. Anna June shared with us how much it meant to her that we were working so hard to help Alzheimer's victims.

Most everyone had arrived a couple of days before we came and had had a great time together. Kim was smart to hold the party in Tahoe. Everyone was eager to make a vacation out of the trip. The morning before, there had been a large brunch for everyone, and after that, they all went to decorate the banquet room. The day following the dinner, there was a picnic at Tahoe's beach. I still can't quite believe that it really happened. I will treasure the memory of that day forever.

Kim organized the whole thing. She felt it was important for all the family to get together, and for all the cousins to see each other again after so many years. All the kids pitched in and helped. Our wedding picture had been enlarged into a large poster. There was a banquet complete with anniversary cake. There was the brunch and picnic. That's a lot to organize. Kim worked on this project for an entire year. I shudder to think of all those phone calls they had to make to keep everyone motivated and the details scheduled. How Kim managed to get all those people, not only to arrange for time off to come, but also to gather up their families to make the trip, still amazes me.

After the kids gave those glowing tributes to me and Johnny, I was moved to tears, but I was also feeling pretty awful because I had said such terrible things about my kids when none of them would come to Tahoe with us. To think that I had complained because they didn't even care enough to even to come to dinner for our anniversary! It serves me right to feel guilty. I felt like an ungrateful witch. I love my kids. I was glad to hear them say they loved and appreciated us, too, and that they know how much Johnny and I love them.

We were given a Caribbean Cruise, and Johnny and I had the time of our lives. There will never be another party like the celebration the kids put on for us for our fortieth anniversary.

Our work with the Alzheimer's Aid Society is rewarding. Johnny and I have been surprised and pleased to have been honored for doing something that is its own reward. When these honors have come our way, it has been hard to believe that it's happening to us.

In 1986, I received the Jefferson Award, which is

sponsored by KOVR-TV in Sacramento, and was initiated in 1976 by Samuel Beard, then an aide of the late Senator Robert Kennedy. Its purpose is to pay tribute to people not ordinarily recognized for their services to their communities. I was pleased to receive this honor, but more than personal satisfaction was the knowledge that work with Alzheimer's victims and caregivers was receiving more attention.

It was a wonderful honor for me to be featured on the 700 Club on national television. And with this recognition, Alzheimer's disease again receives recognition. The more people know of this disease, the more help will become available.

I received the JCPenney Golden Rule Award for Outstanding Volunteer Service. It was hard to believe that all this was happening to me. I sometimes pinch myself to see if it's real.

In 1994, Johnny received the Jefferson Award. When he retired, he took over all the public speaking and training, and has been working more than full time since. In one year, in addition to speaking to service clubs and other groups, he conducted two hundred seventy-five in-services to nursing homes and long-term care facilities. Many nights he comes home so tired he can hardly stand up. But he keeps going. I couldn't do all this without Johnny. We make a good team.

Many articles have been written about us and the Alzheimer's Aid Society. The more recognition Alzheimer's receives, the better service victim's and their caregivers will receive. Five years ago, when I

mentioned Alzheimer's disease, very few people knew
what it was. Some thought it was a memory loss asso-
ciated with old age. Fifteen years ago, no major research
was being done on Alzheimer's disease. Today, medical research centers throughout the country are doing
research on Alzheimer's disease.

Doctors have said to us, "Our job is to find a
cure and prevention, Your job is to help families cope
with the inevitable." Johnny and I hope that the day
will come when our job won't be necessary.

CHAPTER SIXTEEN

Promises To Keep

I have always felt that the greatest tragedy of Alzheimer's disease, and there are so many tragedies, is the loss of a person's dignity. Everything an individual has ever had is gone, taken away by this vicious killer. The victim of Alzheimer's disease is robbed of all that makes a life valuable, of the ability to think, to recognize friends and family, to love and communicate, and to take care of the simplest needs.

Alzheimer's sneaks up on us in unsuspecting ways and moves with painful slowness along its cruel and deadly journey of destruction. Those of us who have lived with this disease cannot help but wonder, when normal confusion enters our lives, if perhaps we are not its next victim. We cringe in fear to think of ourselves in this plight, not only for having to endure this terrible pain and suffering, but for the years of pain and suffering we will cause our families and loved ones.

Alzheimer's disease often begins with the victim becoming generally disoriented. Routine things are forgotten. Difficulty with daily activities develops. Behavior takes disturbing turns. Physical coordination diminishes. Personality changes emerge.

Much of the victim's early behavior is an exaggeration of normal behavior, of the things we all do. We all forget things. We all are irrational at times. We all become impatient and angry. We can all remember feeling disoriented at one time or other. And so we question ourselves when we suspect that something is wrong, while at the same time, we deny the symptoms. We are afraid, and we don't really want to know if this nightmare is happening to us.

Often, in our ignorance, we blame the ones who are struggling with the onset of Alzheimer's. We don't realize they are sick, and we accuse them of being lazy, or careless, or irresponsible, or inconsistent, or forgetful. We are angry because they are difficult and irrational, and we think that they aren't really trying to be better. We don't know that Alzheimer's patients are doing the best they can do. We don't understand that they are more afraid of what's happening than anybody. We don't understand their struggle to remember, to say the right thing, to get things right. We don't know their feelings of isolation when their minds disintegrate as they struggle to hold on.

Alzheimer's is a disease. It is not a matter of aging. My mama and brothers and sisters were afflicted when they were in their early forties. With the exception of Norma Jean, they all died in their early fifties. People can live into their eighties and nineties and still have functional minds. Alzheimer's disease leaves the gray cortex of the brain nerve cells incurably tangled and dysfunctional. It is a disease.

When members of my family were ill with Alzheimer's disease, we were told it was very rare. Today, government statistics tell us that complications from Alzheimer's disease ranks fourth as the leading cause of death in America. Victims of Alzheimer's disease account for about half of the nursing home population. Alzheimer's disease kills about 120,000 people a year. It is not rare.

Not only does the one with Alzheimer's disease need care, the ones caring for that person need help. Providing care to someone who is irrational, hostile, incontinent, and sometimes violent is a most demanding and difficult task. It is fruitless and thankless. There is never a "Thank you," or "I love you." Never a word of appreciation. The disease is relentless. There is no cure. Only death stops Alzheimer's disease.

Alzheimer's disease has been described as a movie of a person's life being run backwards. A person begins with the present and moves step by step back through his life experiences, forgetting each phase forever as he passes through it. But the rewind is distorted. Worn film and torn sprocket holes jolt the pictures erratically. What you see is a life out of focus and distorted. The sound is garbled. Dust has collected on the film, obliterating crucial details. This rewind of a person's life does not go smoothly.

The burdens of caring for an individual ill with Alzheimer's disease are more than physical. They drain the caregiver's emotional and financial reserves as well. Caregivers need a break. They need respite care. They need emotional support. They need support groups. They need education about what is happening. They need financial help. They need services for the victims of the disease.

Often, friends of the caregiver disappear once the behavior of an individual turns erratic. So very often people don't know what to do. They feel awkward and uncomfortable about being around someone who has Alzheimer's disease or even around the caregiver. This leaves the caregiver more alone than ever at a time when friendship is vital.

If you know someone who is a caregiver, call often, spend some time visiting, go to your friend for an afternoon so the caregiver can take a break. Stop by with a casserole for dinner. Take the caregiver out to a movie. And most important, listen so that they can tell of their pain and frustration. Offer a willing hand and a caring heart. What is needed more than anything is support and respite for the caregiver.

Had I not found God on a deep and personal level, I don't believe I could have stood up against the fears and depression that were taking control of my life. God's love has given me the strength and courage to do what I would never have been able to do. I am not a leader by nature. I have a ninth grade education and a few courses at the local college, but I don't have any degrees. I have had to disregard these shortcomings and move forward. This would never have been possible without my deep faith in God.

My promise to God was that I would do whatever I could to help others who were living with the nightmare of Alzheimer's disease. Remembering and renewing my promise help me attend another support group, make another phone call, listen to another person calling out for help, get out another newsletter, and organize another workshop.

Johnny and I work toward helping to educate the public. The more people know about Alzheimer's disease, the more effort will be made toward finding a cure. We also participate and support research. But day in and day out, the backbone of our work is to help caregivers, because caregivers are also victims. The disease ravages their lives emotionally, physically, and financially. It invades their lives for years, causing disruption and chaos, pain and torment, guilt and suffering.

Sometimes, when I am asked once again to go to a medical center to be tested, when I find myself tired of being stuck with needles and crammed into MRI machines, weary of giving blood and skin, and bored from sitting through endless hours of taking psychological tests I have taken a dozen times before, I am tempted, however briefly, not to go.

Then I remember my promise, and I think of Mama and of Herschel and Leonard, of Minnie Sue and Norma Jean. I think of my children and my grandchildren, of my nieces and nephews, and grand nieces and grand nephews. I think of the cruelty of Alzheimer's disease and the haunting possibility that it might strike one of them. And I remember the shining, innocent faces of all the young people and children at our anniversary celebration. I remember their eager expressions as I listened to their dreams of their futures. Then I know I must go whenever and wherever I am called upon to go. And if I have helped, even in the smallest way, I know that my efforts have been more than worth it.

The problems of Alzheimer's disease do not end. That's why our efforts must not end. I am lucky and grateful that Johnny is here hand in hand with me. So many times, his support has kept me going. I keep going, too, because I made a promise to God, and promises are forever.

BOOK TWO

Help for the Caregiver

SHARING IDEAS

People call us for help, for advice, for information, and just to talk with someone who understands. This second section of the book offers information we share regularly with caregivers and their families. Included are case histories. Many of them we have experienced first hand. Others have been shared with us. With those case histories, we include what we and others have done to help ease the suffering of patients as well as to help make the caregiver's task less harrowing.

The First Steps

Get An Accurate Diagnosis

When a person or family calls for the first time and wonders what to do, the first thing we advise them to do is to see a neurologist. The last thing in the world anyone wants to know is that someone in their family has Alzheimer's disease, and we always hope that the person has something else. There are many diseases that mimic Alzheimer's disease which are treatable. As yet, there is no test to determine with complete accuracy whether or not someone is in the beginning stages of Alzheimer's disease, but neurologists can determine with a high degree of accuracy whether or not a person has the disease. There is only one way to find out for sure, and that is by doing an autopsy after the individual has passed away. Researchers now believe that an accurate test will be available within a very few years.

Find Legal Help

If Alzheimer's disease is indicated, we suggest that the family see an attorney who specializes in elder law. They should do this right away. Often immediate steps need to be taken to protect the family as well as the person who is ill. Alzheimer's victims have been known to squander a life's savings before the family knows what is happening. Homes have been lost. It is common for financial responsibility and authority to be transferred out of the hands of the victim and subsequently handled by another family member, a trustee or guardian. Guardianship may be in order. Families are reluctant to take away a patient's legal and financial rights, but the action is often necessary. An attorney who specializes in elder law is knowledgeable in these areas and can advise you.

Help for Caregivers

Over the years, Johnny and I have been blessed to know hundreds of kind and loving people who have lived with and cared for a family member with Alzheimer's disease. We have listened to their stories and shared our experiences, hoping to make their lives a little easier. This sharing of ideas and experiences has been a two-way street. These courageous and creative people have provided us with many valuable lessons. With sincere thanks to all of them, we share many of these ideas with you. First, however, a few words of caution are necessary:

> **There are no easy answers. Nothing works all of the time. Some things will work for one person and not for another. If something works, relish the moment. It may never work again. Sometimes, nothing seems to help.**
>
> **Johnny and I know that these suggestions for caregivers have worked some of the time for some individuals. Some of these ideas have worked often with many.**
>
> **We offer these suggestions in the hope that at least some of them will help you. There are no guarantees, but we believe they are certainly worth a try.**

Four Cardinal Rules

Cardinal Rule One:

Remember that the people who have Alzheimer's disease are giving everything they have to give. They are trying as hard as they can. They are doing the best they can do. They are giving one hundred per cent of what they are capable of giving. A person with Alzheimer's disease is suffering from fear and loneliness as the mind drifts out of control and their world disintegrates. This individual wants and needs your approval.

Cardinal Rule Two:

Remember to be loving and kind because it will make life less difficult for the Alzheimer's victim <u>and for you</u>. Those with Alzheimer's disease need love and understanding, too. A smile, a laugh, a hug, or a gentle touch can go a long way toward providing good care.
Remember to:

> Talk softly; try not to shout or yell.
> Encourage; try not to criticize or scold.
> Be gentle; try not to be harsh.
> Listen; try not to argue.
> Suggest alternatives; try not to tell the person, "No."
> Agree with the individual whenever possible.

It is pointless and cruel to punish a person who has Alzheimer's disease. It may sound as though we are suggesting that the caregivers do the impossible. We know that people with Alzheimer's disease are terribly difficult to manage. Losing your temper or patience will only make it worse. Providing good care will make your task less difficult. I don't say, "Make the task easier," because being a caregiver of an individual who has Alzheimer's disease is never easy.

Nobody can be patient all the time. When you lose it, admit it. Try to laugh at your lapses. Know that everyone has them. Don't blame yourself. Put the unfortunate incident behind you and go on

Cardinal Rule Three:

Divert the patient's attention. In real estate, there are three things to remember: location, location, and location. With an Alzheimer's victim, there are also three things to remember: diversion, diversion, and diversion.

Think of an alternative. Offer a new activity. Change the subject. Ask a question. Bribe or lie a little if necessary. You may find it shocking that a Christian woman would tell you to do such things, but I do. If helping an individual means "bribing" them with a new activity or a cookie, do it. If it takes telling a "little white lie," tell it. Do it and don't feel guilty. Suggest going fishing tomorrow. Or shopping. Offer to do something special. The person with Alzheimer's disease will never remember. Offer a treat. If a bribe works, use it.

Cardinal Rule Four:

Remember to take care of the caregiver. If you are the caregiver, take care of yourself. If you know a caregiver, offer and give help. A caregiver's task is an impossible one.

It helps if all family members are involved. Wherever possible, insist that each takes turns on a regular basis to relieve the primary caregiver. It not only makes things easier for the primary caregiver, it helps other family members understand the problems more clearly. We can't stress how important it is to have as many family members as possible involved with the care of the one who has Alzheimer's disease. If you are the primary caregiver, don't try to do it all alone. If there are no family members available, look elsewhere for help. Find where you can get some help and relief. Don't try to do it all by yourself.

Locate day care facilities in your area.
Call on friends and relatives to help.
Call your local senior service office.
Call on your minister or priest.
Attend a support group for caregivers.

Make a list of things others can do to help you. When people ask what they can do to help, tell them. Give them the list and let them choose. You are facing a crisis. This is not the time to be shy.

Disregard criticism from friends and relatives who find fault with everything you do. Every family has at least one and sometimes more. Give the critic a turn at caring for the Alzheimer's victim while you cultivate supportive relationships. Support groups are filled with others who understand what you are going through and need your friendship in the same way you need theirs.

Alzheimer's Disease is More than a Memory Loss

The common perception that Alzheimer's disease only causes memory loss in very old people is inaccurate. Alzheimer's disease usually occurs in older people, but it can strike individuals in their forties or fifties, and it is vastly more than a memory loss.

It is a once reasonable person who hoards bits of paper and hides things. It is a once vital, interested person who stares blankly at nothing. It is a once responsible person who no longer can make the simplest decisions. It is a once articulate person who mumbles incoherently. It is a once trusting person who has become obsessed and paranoid. It is a once loving person who now screams and swears angrily. It is a once fastidious person who no longer bathes or can use the bathroom. It is a once conversational person who repeats meaningless words or sentences over and over and over. It is a once gentle person who has become violent.

Caring for someone who has this terrible disease is an endless, difficult, tiring, discouraging, thankless, and challenging job. It is feeding a person who refuses to eat. It is diapering an incontinent adult six or seven times a day. It is caring for someone who no longer knows who you are. It is a life on rewind. It is a movie run backward, but without balance or reason. Alzheimer's disease is vastly more than a memory loss. Those of you who are caregivers already know that.

Life on the Rewind Cycle

Johnny and I first heard of Alzheimer's disease described as a person's life being run backward like a film or video being rewound from Dr. Charles Borowiak, head of the Department of Gerontology at American River College. The Alzheimer's disease patients begin by being forgetful and disoriented and move backward through their lives. The journey does not go smoothly. The final stage of the disease is complete helplessness, often ending with the person curled into the fetal position.

The idea of Alzheimer's disease as the rewinding of a person's life gave us new insight that helped us help others. Now, we always try to find out as much as we can about the life of the person who has Alzheimer's disease. This "life history" information can help the family anticipate and understand the erratic behaviors they will face and have to cope with as the disease progresses.

With Alzheimer's disease, short term memory disappears right away. The long term memory remains intact for a longer time. A person with Alzheimer's disease can remember what happened to them at six or sixteen, but can't remember what was said or what happened six minutes ago.

Dr. Borowiak's illustration has proven accurate again and again. After each phase of life is reenacted in this rewinding of the tape of life, the memory of that period of time fades and disappears. For example, a person who spoke a different language as a child, and who learned English as an adult, will eventually forget how to speak English, but may remember the first language. That person has moved backward through life until reaching the time before he learned English. All memory of speaking English will have been erased. After not speaking for a period of time, patients have been known to chatter ecstatically when spoken to in their original language.

Johnny was visiting a care center where two Croatian patients had not spoken for months. Johnny, whose family spoke Croatian when he was a child, spoke to them, asking, "How are you?" in Croatian. Their faces lit up, and they began talking away in their native language. Johnny had long since forgotten most of the Croatian he had learned as a child and couldn't understand a word they were saying. He just smiled and nodded. The two Croatian men were so busy talking away they didn't seem to notice or care that Johnny wasn't part of their conversation.

Another time, Johnny and I came across this woman named Rose who had worked in her church for almost twenty years before developing Alzheimer's disease. To everyone's surprise and embarrassment, she began cursing. People coming into the church for the first time questioned whether they wanted to come back. In checking with Rose's family, we learned that, in her early twenties, she worked as a bar maid where swearing was common place.

A gentleman named Charles suffered from Alzheimer's disease and one day out of the blue, he started spitting everywhere. Nobody could understand why. He didn't seem to be angry at anybody. He just spit all the time. He spit when he was walking down the hall. He would spit when his wife took him out for dinner to a restaurant. The other diners weren't very happy about it. After a few choice splats on the carpet, the manager invariably asked them to leave. Charles would stand in the middle of a room and spit over and over again. His wife Ethel did her best to keep him in the kitchen where mopping up was easier. She was completely confused and not very happy with her husband's new hobby.

When she asked Johnny for help, the first thing he did was contact Charles' family and found that Charles had grown up on a farm. His brother remembered that Charles had been in a spitting contest when he was about twelve and had evidently done quite well. Charles had practiced for that contest for weeks, spitting all of the time everywhere.

Johnny told Ethel he thought that, by the time Charles regressed beyond the age of twelve, the spitting would stop. Shortly afterward it did.

We were visiting Harlan, a caregiver, and his wife Mary. We found Mary sitting in a rocker pretending to nurse a doll. She had twelve children and had nursed all of them. She had regressed to the time in her life where she was nursing one of her babies and seemed to have found contentment and satisfaction in "nursing" a doll. Since she had had so many children, this stage would probably last a fairly long time.

Mary would hold the doll to her breast while she rocked back and forth, humming soothingly to her "baby." Harlan said that sometimes she would wake him in the middle of the night and tell him to go get some food for the "baby." Harlan would tell her that he already got the food and would go back to sleep. For the most part, Mary's activity didn't cause any problem, except that her family had stopped taking her out in public. No matter where she went, she would bare her breast and nurse her doll.

I remember my sister Norma Jean telling me that she wanted to go upstairs to bed. She lived in a one story home in Southern California and had lived there for years. That house didn't have an upstairs, but in the house where we grew up on Reynolds Street in Kansas City, the bedrooms were upstairs.

Mae couldn't understand why all of a sudden her mother, who had Alzheimer's disease, had become constantly irritable with her. They had been close friends for the last twenty years. During questioning, it came out that Mae had been a challenging and re-bellious teenager, giving her mother a very bad time. Evidently, her mother had regressed to this period and was reenacting her relationship with her troublesome daughter.

This hostile behavior would probably continue until the mother had lived through those difficult years, but now Mae had a better understanding of what was happening and was able to be more patient with her cranky mother. This stage, too, would pass.

Jim spent his days in the nursing home walking along the halls running his hands along the surface of the walls. He had been a plasterer and was checking to see if the wall was smooth.

A nun continually approached staff members and, handing them a rolled up towel, asked them to give it to the doctor. She had been a nurse in her younger years. Another retired nurse with Alzheimer's wrapped feces in Kleenex and told everyone she was saving them for the doctor.

Lucille spent her days in the nursing home pacing the halls and repeating, "Mom, why don't you believe me. Why don't you believe me." It turned out that Lucille had been molested when she was twelve.

A retired executive sits all day and cracks walnuts. As a boy he shelled walnuts and sold the nut meats for spending money. Bring the man more walnuts to crack until this phase passes.

If the behavior is harmless, let it be. Don't debate the issue with an individual who has Alzheimer's disease. It is a waste of time to try to be rational. It is pointless to discourage them. If a person is not hurting anybody or anything, think of the activity as a blessing that keeps the person busy and entertained. If a person is content living through earlier years, be thankful the individual has found comfort.

If the activity is harmful, try diversion. Offer a cookie, suggest joining you for a walk outside, or turn on the television set. <u>Do not hesitate to ask for help if you need it.</u>

It is important to learn about the victims' lives. It is common for a person who is the oldest or youngest in the family, or is an only child, to be especially difficult. An only child is often used to getting his way, and with the illness, this spoiled-child behavior intensifies. Tantrums and pouting are common. Oldest children are used to being bossy and controlling their younger brothers and sisters. When they become ill with Alzheimer's disease, they tend to be controlling and bossy. The only girl in a large family of boys, or the only boy in a large family of girls, often received special treatment as children. When ill, they often demand and expect to be treated better than those around them. They expect to be pampered.

Learn if the individual's family had few or many children, whether the person lived in the city, in a small town, or on a farm. A person raised on a farm many years ago may not recognize an indoor bathroom and be looking for an outhouse. What was the family's financial status? What were the person's interests? What was the person's professional background or work history? Understanding an individual's background can provide clues to help the caregiver cope with what seems to be totally irrational behavior.

Understanding that the individual is living in a different time will ease the pain of not being recognized as the wife or husband or child. The person with Alzheimer's disease might say, "You're not my wife.

You're too old." In the patient's eyes, he is married to the twenty-your-old he married fifty or sixty years ago.

Knowing the patient's background will not change the patient's behavior. Knowing the patient's family history can help the caregiver understand the patient's behavior. Understanding why a person is doing something can relieve some of the caregiver's anxiety and worry. It can help caregivers be more accepting of an individual's seemingly endless array of crazy antics, and it can give the caregiver the opportunity to find creative approaches for dealing with undesirable behavior.

Some Typical Behaviors

The Desire To Please

While each person is different and has different experiences, many behaviors are common to most Alzheimer's patients. The patients usually know something is wrong and that, as hard as they try, they are not going to get it right. They are often frightened and sometimes angry. Refusal to do something may be due more to fear of failure than to being stubborn.

Victims of Alzheimer's disease see the caregivers as their security, and they follow the caregiver everywhere. This is called "shadowing" and can drive the caregiver bonkers. A person with Alzheimer's disease tries to be helpful, and their efforts can also be upsetting to the caregiver. I can think of two perfect examples of the desire to please gone awry.

Our friend Irene loved to garden. Tending her flowers provided relaxing therapy and helped her handle the stress of caring for her husband Edwin. One day as she finished planting and weeding, she asked Edwin to bring in her tools for her. Irene went on into the house. Edwin cheerfully complied. Not only did he bring in the tools, he went the extra mile and did more for Irene. He pulled up all the plants she had just planted and brought them in along with the tools. He wanted to give her a special gift. He wanted to please her. Sometimes it is very hard to show your appreciation!

Jane was busily fixing lunch when the door bell rang. She asked her husband Frank to help her and please open a can of tuna as she went to the door. Then the phone rang. When she finally went back into the kitchen, she found that Frank had helped a lot. He had proceeded to open up all the cans he could find. Olives, a two-pound can of coffee, applesauce, tomato sauce, smoked clams, a very expensive small can of truffles imported from France that Jane was saving for a special occasion, V8 juice, green beans, beets, peaches, you name it. He smiled at his wife, pleased with himself that he had done so well and been so helpful. At a time like this, it is difficult to be appreciative. It was a struggle for Jane to say, "Thank you."

Hiding Things

Anyone who has spent much time with a person who has Alzheimer's disease can tell stories of how patients routinely hide things. The elderly of today grew up at a time when it was common for people to put money under the mattress, or behind the cookie jar, or in a sugar bowl. On more than one occasion, I have located coins and dollar bills pushed down into a sugar bowl. It makes for a sticky mess.

Many of today's Alzheimer's patients were young adults during the great depression when there was a widespread distrust of banks. It was common practice for folks to hide their money and other valuables for safekeeping. Under the mattress was a favorite spot. An intruder would have to wake them up to get at their savings.

We know of two cases where, after Alzheimer's patients had died, family members were cleaning out their homes. When the trash cans were emptied, $40,000 was found at the bottom of one and over $20,000 at the bottom of another. If you are caring for an Alzheimer's victim, for heaven's sakes, never throw out the trash, or anything else for that matter, without checking very thoroughly and carefully to see what treasures might be hidden there.

When a caregiver called to tell us that she gives her mother two dollars every day, and although her mother never leaves the house, no one knows what happens to the money. Johnny suggested she put the phone receiver down and go immediately and look under the mattress. We heard a squeal of delight. Sure enough, there was the stash of one dollar bills.

When a visiting nurse who cares for an individual who has Alzheimer's disease called me, she was very concerned. A treasured and very valuable family ring was missing, and the husband had confronted the nurse, suspecting that she had taken it. She was advised to look under the mattress. It was there. The husband was embarrassed for having accused the nurse. The nurse was relieved to be cleared of any wrongdoing.

Gifts, pieces of clothing, reading glasses, treasured family pictures, as well as odds and ends and bits of junk are regularly stowed away for safe keeping. One individual made a practice of putting uneaten food under her bed. The smell of old tuna sandwiches and rotting orange slices helped track down the problem, but not everything is so easily located. Make a habit of checking out-of-the-way places. Looking behind the dresser or couch might yield a cache of hidden valuables. One person hid things in the back of the closet. Another continually stashed her treasures in the dirty clothes basket. A good place to start looking, however, is under the mattress. That seems to be the number-one, favorite spot.

Hallucination and Delusion

It is not uncommon for a person with Alzheimer's disease to see things that aren't there. If Dad sees animals on the wall or ceiling, never tell him there aren't any animals there. Say something like,

"Dad, I know you see them, but I don't." When Jenny sees a man under her bed, try talking to her about him. If the individual is not frightened by the hallucinations, don't worry about them. When the hallucinations are frightening, calm the person and divert his attention. Don't argue or try to explain. Logic is useless. Forget it. Discuss the hallucinations in conversation or distract the person. It sometimes helps to involve the person. If there are bugs on the floor, let the person help vacuum them up. Then divert attention with a snack or other activity.

Often a person will see one thing and think it is something else. I watched a man pick up a slice of white bread and use it to blow his nose. He obviously thought the bread was a handkerchief. The flowers in the wall paper pattern must be picked. The image in the mirror is another person. This person can be a new friend or a dangerous stranger. A polished floor can be seen as water. A person ill with Alzheimer's disease may fear falling in and drowning. Different colored tiles on the floor may be seen as holes, and the individual may fear falling into one of them. If the patient is afraid, the fear is real. Don't make light of it. Physical symptoms of fear are common. The frightened person will perspire, the heart rate will increase, and breathing will become rapid. Sometimes, a person will shake from fear. Comfort and calm that individual as you would a frightened child. Then use diversion.

Repetition, Pacing, and Compulsive Behavior

Restlessness and repeated behaviors drive caregivers up the wall. Individuals will repeat behaviors over and over and over. Try not to let it drive you batty. Ignore the behavior that isn't dangerous or destructive. When an individual with Alzheimer's disease tells the same story for the thousandth time, nod and smile as you try and let it go in one ear and out the other. There is nothing you can do about it anyway. The person will pace back and forth, back and forth. Think of all the good exercise the individual is getting. Living with Alzheimer's disease is a challenge. It helps if the caregiver can look at the positive side.

Changes in Personal Hygiene

It is typical for those with Alzheimer's disease who had always been clean and neat before they became ill to become careless about personal cleanliness. Those with Alzheimer's disease often resist what were once routine habits of keeping clean. They don't want to wash their faces and hands, brush their teeth, or comb their hair. They have been known to go take a shower and come back still dirty and with a dry towel. I sometimes wonder if they are pulling a stunt they pulled as kids, or if they have just forgotten what they had set out to do? Either way, don't be cross. Try again. Use a different approach. You may have to take the individual to the shower or help wash dirty hands. You may have to overlook a little dirt.

Victims have been known to complain that the bath water is cold when it is not cold at all. Years ago in rural areas, by the time child number three or four or five got a turn in the tub, the water would indeed be cold. It would not only be cold, it would be dirty. When they tell you the water is cold or dirty, they probably can't tell the difference between bath time today and bath time sixty-five years ago.

A major problem for caregivers is to get their loved one to take a bath. He or she could well be reverting to childhood days. Children, too, often resist. Begin by removing the person's clothing slowly and gently, talking in a soothing way all the time. It doesn't always work, but it works more often and much more effectively than being stern and ordering someone who is ill to take a bath. I've heard individuals scream as though they were being tortured while refusing to put a toe in the water. It's no wonder caregivers learn to live with a little dirt behind the ears.

Years ago, Saturday night was bath night. Try telling the patient that it's Saturday night already and time for a bath. It doesn't matter that it is Wednesday. If it works, use the same story on Thursday. The patient will never know the difference.

Try giving an old fashioned, spit bath. Don't use spit, of course. Use a warm, damp wash cloth and go after the most offending spots of dirt. The surgeon general isn't coming by to do an inspection. Remember to talk quietly or hum softly while accomplishing the task of washing.

Sometimes men resist being bathed by other men. As children, their mothers bathed them. Years ago, most fathers did not bathe their children. Caregivers have also found that women are easier to diaper than men. Women wore sanitary napkins. Men did not, and they rebel more often at being diapered.

Some individuals love taking a bath or shower. Getting them out of the tub or stall becomes the problem. Try bribery! Offer a special game or favorite treat. Keep a person clean enough to be sanitary, but relax a little. Don't strive for perfection!

Changes in Eating Habits

Sooner or later, most people suffering from Alzheimer's disease have difficulty eating. Often an individual refuses to eat, or after eating willingly for some time, suddenly stops. Sometimes the person is so confused he or she cannot decide which food on the plate to eat. It is often helpful to serve one kind of food on the plate at a time. Provide only one utensil. Clear the table of other distractions. Provide the least confusion possible at meal time.

Breakfast is often the main meal of the day. If the individual finishes everything on the plate, offer another item, such as a piece of toast or fruit. Fruit juice is popular for breakfast. Provide a multivitamin daily. With changes in eating and exercise patterns, many will benefit from a stool softener. Just remember to promote adequate fluid intake when you are giving stool softeners. If water is rejected, give juice or jello.

Try not to present individuals who have Alzheimer's disease with a situation that requires making a decision. Do not ask what kind of soup they would like. Do not ask if they prefer soup or a sandwich. You may be trying to be considerate, but by asking, you are only making life more difficult. If you are at a restaurant, do not ask what the Alzheimer's victim would like to order. You order.

One caregiver called, frustrated that his wife could never make up her mind about what she wanted to eat. His solution was to take her to a buffet. This was the worst possible thing he could have done. The outing was a disaster. Since that caregiver told me about taking his wife to a buffet, I have come across others who have done the same thing. They thought buffet style or cafeteria style dining was the solution for those who can't decide. Please don't take individuals who suffer from Alzheimer's disease out to eat where they have to make multiple decisions. Forget the buffet. Stick with a tuna sandwich or bowl of soup.

The difficulty of decision making extends beyond choosing which food to eat. Don't ask a person who is confused to choose a table. Don't think you are being thoughtful if you ask. "Where would you like to sit?" The table settings in many restaurants include too many things. A vase of flowers, water glasses and wine glasses, dinner forks and salad forks, plates and salad plates, salt, pepper and sugar. Quickly and quietly remove as many things as you can.

People walking by the table or talking at the surrounding tables contribute to the overall chaos for the Alzheimer's victim. When dining out, select the restaurant with care.

All dinnerware should be plain. Designs of any kind can be distracting. Sometimes an individual will confuse the patterns with something to eat.

Provide a plain table cover. Flowered or printed table coverings cause confusion. People have been known to try to eat the flowers or pick off the designs.

Provide one bowl, or plate. Provide a spoon or fork, never both.

Put a drop of food coloring in a glass of water. This makes the water visible, and the patient can tell if they have water or not.

Cut food into bite sized pieces.

Provide finger food.

Tuna or peanut-butter-and-jelly sandwiches are usually a hit. They are kid's favorites today and were kid's favorites a long time ago. Muffins, on the other hand, are less popular. Many care facilities have tried both and find that the sandwiches are the big winners. It is interesting to note that, even years ago, many more children liked tuna or peanut butter sandwiches than liked muffins.

It is not uncommon for individuals to forget that they have eaten and request a second or third meal. After eating a meal, a person will often complain that nobody feeds them.

Jim was in a care home and when visited by his sister, told her that he had not eaten. She went immediately to find him something to eat. Jim's wife arrived about thirty minutes later. Jim told her that he hadn't eaten. She arranged for him to have breakfast. She then went to the staff to complain. When the aide checked his chart, she noted that he had eaten breakfast three times, one when everyone was eating, another provided by his sister, and finally the meal his wife got for him.

Use diversion. Say that lunch was delicious, and then distract the individual. Do not, in any circumstances, argue and insist that you know full well that they have eaten and prove your point by telling them in detail what they ate. They won't remember. Besides, winning a debate with someone who has Alzheimer's disease is not a significant accomplishment.

Know that the day will come when a person ill with Alzheimer's disease will need help eating. Feeding an individual who is ill is a common task of caregivers.

Changes in Sleeping Habits

You will wonder what happened to regular hours. The internal clocks of individuals with Alzheimer's disease are frequently out of whack, often disrupting entire households. Try to see to it that the individual has plenty of exercise during the day. Being physically tired by nightfall sometimes helps a person fall asleep. If an individual wants to sleep on the couch or in a favorite chair, don't make an issue out of it. If the desire is to sleep in regular clothing rather than in pajamas, so be it. There are plenty of other things to worry about.

If you are unable to get an individual to bed and to sleep at a decent hour, or if the individual wakes up at all hours of the night, make sure the house and yard are secure and adequately lighted. One can wander safely if areas are secure. Some people will listen to music or watch television. As long as the person is safe and not demanding your attention, you can get some sleep.

Paranoia

Know that when your loved one starts accusing you of stealing, you are not alone. Paranoia is a common trait of people with Alzheimer's disease. Don't take the accusations personally. Caregivers and other family members are often accused of stealing. Help the individual look for the lost item. Distract the individual as soon as possible. If you don't, it is not uncommon for a person to rant on and on ad nauseam. It's futile to argue and declare your innocence. Divert the individual's attention. Sometimes that's the only way you're going to get off the hook!

We know victims who have accused their caregivers and friends of stealing their money and their belongings. They have accused spouses of infidelity.

They are convinced that someone is spying on them or planning to hurt them. Paranoia is one of the more difficult and unpleasant aspects of Alzheimer's disease. If someone complains of being mistreated, it won't help to tell that person he is being silly. Check into the allegations. Occasionally, those complaints are true. If you find no cause for concern, explain matter-of-factly that the thief, or mugger, or adulterer, who ever the culprit is, won't do it again. Then distract the individual. Try not to dwell on the persistent paranoia. Unfair accusations can wear down any of us.

Alzheimer's victims have been known to threaten to harm their caregivers if they don't stop committing some imagined offense. Such threats often come at a time when the victim no longer recognizes the caregiver.

If the threats and accusations are directed at you, try not to take them personally. It is important to keep a balance. If at all possible, keep a sense of humor. After all, the accusations are laughable. One eighty-year-old caregiver, whose husband was accusing her of having a young boyfriend, explained to us that she hadn't found him yet, but if we would keep our eyes open for him, she would appreciate it. She definitely had things in perspective. Don't take yourself too seriously.

Aggression and Violence

If a person becomes violent, it is time to get help. Perhaps the most difficult aspect of Alzheimer's disease is the aggressive and even violent behavior of a loved one. A once gentle and caring mother, father, husband or wife turns angry. Seemingly illogical combativeness can lead to violence. Caregivers can be hurt. Johnny and I believe that when a person becomes unruly and violent, it is time to consider placement in a care facility. The staff there is trained to manage aggressive individuals. The family is not. Often the caregiver is elderly and not physically able to protect him or herself.

Those with Alzheimer's disease are no longer in control of their lives. Others tell them what to do and when to do it. Fears mount. Frustration builds. Some individuals resent being under the control of women who make up most of the staff of care facilities. Others resent being under the control of men who make up most of the medical profession. Wherever possible, a balance should be reached so that opportunities exists for relating to both men and women in a caregiver situation. Physicians can prescribe medication to ease some of the aggression. The caregiver's pain of being on the receiving end of verbal and physical abuse is devastating. No one should be subjected to dangerous and painful attack. When aggression takes over, seek help. It is time for placement in a long-term care facility.

People are reluctant to admit it could happen to them. They don't want the world to know that their beloved Sam or Mary is striking out at them or swearing at them. It is only natural for caregivers not to want to admit that their loved ones are accusing them of doing all kinds of terrible things. Pride is a factor. Loyalty is a factor.

Safety is also a factor. It's time to seek help.

Changes in Sexual Behavior

It is not uncommon for a father to become sexually aggressive with his daughter, confusing her with his wife. The same is true with mothers becoming aggressive with their sons. Men have been known to demand sexual activity five and six times a day. Remember that the short term memory is gone. Explain briefly that you have just had sex and it was wonderful. Immediately divert the individual's attention to something else. Candy bars are a favorite with Alzheimer's patients. Have a handy supply of miniature bars.

With some individuals, the duration of excessive sexual activity is short lived, and the person settles down into a non-demanding period. Diversion is the most effective tool, but if nothing distracts the individual from making sexual demands, see your physician about medication. Sexual aggression is disturbing, and if it can not be controlled, Johnny and I believe that it is time for that person to be placed in the hands of professionals.

Thoughts of Suicide

At the onset of Alzheimer's disease, when victims are aware that their minds are twisting out of control, their fear can be devastating. Thoughts of ending their suffering are common. Individuals may talk of "Going into the clouds," or "It's time to go see my mother in Heaven," or "I must find a quiet, restful place." The words are different, but the message is all too familiar. An outing can provide the setting for a person's suicide fantasy. Ways to escape the horror of this destructive disease are appealing. A sailing outing might elicit the comment, "I could slip into the water and never have to live again." A high window might trigger the comment, "I could just float right down." Many think the thoughts. Some succeed in acting on them. It is not unreasonable or uncommon for a caregiver to sympathize with the individual's desperation. The caregiver is powerless to stem the onslaught of the disease. The only options for the caregiver are to make sure the individual is in secure surroundings and to provide as loving and compassionate care as possible. The caregiver needs loving support, too.

General Suggestions

The Magic Touch

Touch is the least expensive, most effective, nonprescription, treatment around. A hug. A touch on the shoulder. A holding of the hand. A back rub. A foot massage. All are messages of love and caring. Use them freely. People with Alzheimer's disease need physical contact, too. Don't be offended by inept overtures for affection. Respond with calm, gentle, reassuring, appropriate contact. For frightened victims, look them in the eye and ask if it is all right for you to give them a hug.

Humor

Humor is another tool that costs nothing and returns much. Laugh in fun, never at a person. Make light of errors. Humor can defuse tension, create camaraderie, and send a message of acceptance and love. Use it freely.

Family Photos

When placing pictures in the rooms of those with Alzheimer's disease, use pictures of family when they were young. An elderly man's wife brought a picture of their fiftieth wedding anniversary. The man was displeased. He wasn't married to that old woman and didn't want anything to do with her. She replaced it with pictures taken on their wedding day. He was pleased with his eighteen-year-old bride.

The use of photos to identify individual's rooms can backfire. Current pictures can be rejected as being too old. The person is now reliving a more youthful time and doesn't want old people around. Sometimes they do not recognize pictures of themselves. One woman became angry at the young woman's face displayed on her door. She was sure it was a woman her husband had been dating and was very definite in her request that the picture be removed immediately. She didn't recognize herself. Win some. Lose some. If something doesn't work, try something else.

Simplify Your Life

Be reasonable in your expectations. Stress and anxiety result in unseemly behavior. Make life easier on yourself. Put unnecessary things away in a high cupboard or packed away in a sealed box. Knick-knacks, extra dishes and cooking utensils, vases, even extra towels and wash cloths can be put out of reach. Remove clothing that is no longer worn. The fewer things there are to lose or hide, the better. Fewer things make for fewer choices.

Make the environment safe. Keep night lights in all rooms where the individual might wander at night. Remove area rugs that might slip. Keep secure locks on all doors to prevent individuals from wandering outside or into off-limits areas. If the yard is securely enclosed, a person may go outside without fear of wandering off and getting lost. If an individual likes to walk in the yard at night, be sure the area has adequate lighting.

Stay with someone who is cooking. Forgetting to watch the pot is common. Things will boil over or burn. A pot holder or dish towel may be set down on a flaming burner. Sharp knives can cause severe wounds. Hot ovens and hot skillets can burn. Dangerous activities must be team activities.

Clothing

Eliminate clothing that is hard to put on and take off. Stick with simple things like jogging suits or sweat suits. They are comfortable, come in a great selection of colors, and can be worn by both men and women. Use pants with elastic waists and shirts that slip easily over the head or button in the front. If a person has a favorite outfit, try to duplicate it. Wearing favorite clothes makes changing easier. Use clothes that are easy to launder and require no ironing. Shoes should be comfortable and easy to get on and off.

Sometimes individuals resist changing into pajamas or night gowns at bed time. If changing into a fresh daytime outfit and letting the individual wear it to bed makes the person happier, do it.

In come cases, nudity can be a problem. Individuals who have Alzheimer's disease have been known to remove their clothing at the most inappropriate times. One man was found outside without a stitch of clothing. When confronted, he replied in a rather childlike voice, "Suzy does it." Suzy was his three-year-old granddaughter.

If you find an individual outside in the buff, gently try leading the person into the house. Take a robe with you and see if you can get the person covered, if not fully dressed. Neighbors will very likely call the police if you leave him outside in his birthday suit. Entice the individual with cookies, candy, or ice cream if necessary.

The other side of the coin is the individual who refuses to remove clothing, especially at bath time, or to change for bed, or to go on an outing. Try diversion. Remember bribery. "Let's change this shirt and then we can have a piece of candy." Or you can give a small treat while attempting to change the person's clothing.

What To Do about Driving the Car

Those of you who have driven with someone who has Alzheimer's disease know how scary that can be. All too often, individuals are allowed to drive long after they are safe. They lose their ability to drive before they lose their desire to drive. You can count on it. We all know that someone who can't remember the rules of the road and who can no longer use good judgment shouldn't be driving a car. We also know, that too many who shouldn't be driving are still on the road.

Replace the car keys with ones that don't fit the ignition, or will go in the ignition, but not turn the starter. Someone with Alzheimer's disease will sometimes fiddle for hours trying to start up the car.

Remove the distributor cap. Disconnect a wire on the starter. The car will not start, and you can sympathize. You can also be sure that nobody is going to be driving anywhere. Keep your keys out of reach.

Sometimes local police will take a person's driver's license away, but all too often, the person with Alzheimer's disease won't care a whit about a license. It is much safer to change keys or dismantle the car.

If public transportation is available, sell the car and save on auto expenses, such as fuel, maintenance, and insurance. Use that money to take a cab in an emergency.

Recently, a visiting nurse took a gentleman who has Alzheimer's disease to the corner coffee shop. She drove his car. When they started home, the victim insisted on driving. Remembering something Johnny had said, the quick-thinking nurse handed the man her own car keys. After struggling for awhile and being unable to get the keys in the ignition, the victim moved into the passenger seat and waited quietly for the nurse to drive him home. The nurse called us to share her success. "It really works," she declared. "It really works."

When Smoking Is a Problem

Among individuals with Alzheimer's disease, there are more men than women who smoke. When these people were young, few women smoked. That will change as new generations become ill, since today, more women than men are starting the habit. If a smoker is not a danger to anyone, let it go. Smoking may well be one of few pleasures the individual still enjoys. In care facilities, there often is a designated area for taking a "smoke break."

If smoking is a problem, however, here is an idea that might help. For the person who has become forgetful about putting down burning cigarettes and creating a safety hazard, give the smoker a pen light for "lighting up." People with Alzheimer's disease are often hesitant to admit failure, and will try over and over before finally giving up.

We came across one woman with Alzheimer's disease who was a heavy smoker, and she was leaving a trail of lighted cigarettes wherever she dropped them or put them down. It didn't matter to her if it was on the kitchen table, the bed, the carpet, or the sofa. Her daughter watched the mother closely, but was panicked that she would miss a burning cigarette, and their house would go up in flames. She tried taking the cigarettes away, but her mother threw tantrums.

Johnny gave the daughter a pen light flashlight and suggested she give it to her mother to use as a cigarette lighter. The mother tried and tried to light up and was unsuccessful. She would not admit failure to her daughter. Much to the daughter's surprise and delight, in about three days, the mother gave up smoking.

Uniforms and People in Positions of Authority

Years ago, people in uniforms were respected. That is not particularly so today. Many afflicted with Alzheimer's disease have regressed to a time when they remember people in uniform to be special. Police officers, firemen, soldiers, priests, nuns, doctors, and nurses were treated with respect. As a rule, the police or paramedics will receive more cooperation than the caregiver will.

If an individual is resisting everything you try

to do, try putting on a uniform. Nursing uniforms are easy to come by, and white clothing might help in a pinch. If you can get your hands on an old stethoscope, do so. We've seen it work on several occasions.

One person we know had an old Naval officer's coat with stripes and all. It worked fine! Turn a white collar around and put on a dark coat. It's worth a try. These suggestions may seem far out, but when you are dealing with a defiant person, they can make a lot of sense.

Bill was having a tantrum and began throwing things around the house. When his wife tried to control him, he turned on her and tried to hit her. Terrified, she quickly called the police. When they arrived, Bill took the officer's hand and went with him as calmly and cooperatively as can be.

Joanne, a registered nurse, always visited her mother on her way home from the hospital and therefore, she was always still wearing her nursing uniform. One Saturday she visited wearing street clothes. Her mother was very hostile. She had recognized the uniform, not the person wearing it.

Fatigue

A tired person is a more difficult person. Morning hours are the best for most people. Late in the day, fatigue plays a major role in a patient's actions and reactions. This "late-in-the-day" fatigue is known as "sundowning." Many individuals suffering with

Alzheimer's disease will become agitated as they tire. An afternoon quiet time from about 2 to 3 o'clock is beneficial. Provide a quiet, calm, peaceful time. Dim the lights. Shut off the phone. Play soft music.

When Mom is caring for Dad, and the kids drop by for a visit, Dad will often be on his best behavior. Alzheimer's victims have a way of rallying for a short period. They can appear quite normal. The kids wonder if anything is really wrong with Dad after all. They think that Mom might be the problem. Those kids need to come back later when Dad falls apart. The individual becomes tired in the late afternoon or evening. If the kids come back when Dad is tired, they will have a much better understanding of what Mom is really going through.

The same scenario can take place when guests arrive. Those with Alzheimer's disease can be charming. They seem to save up their good behavior for company. They invariably put their "best foot forward." When the guests have gone, individuals revert to their trying, exasperating behavior. The guest can't believe that a person is all that difficult and questions the caregiver's assessment. The caregiver is made to feel unreliable. Guilt and self doubt are quick to move in.

Remember, you are the one with the afflicted individual day in and day out. You are the one who knows how that person behaves. Don't let others who have not walked in your shoes drag you down. Invite the skeptic back to care for the individual for a day or two. He or she could use the education. You could use the rest.

When you notice someone becoming tired, frustrated, or anxious, it helps to say that you are tired and want to rest for a little while. Rest together. Avoid becoming tired whenever possible. Break tasks and activities down into small units.

Many individuals find it soothing to have the caregiver read to them from the Bible. Talking books are another source of calming activity, if the content is not too intense. Relaxation tapes can help a person relax and rest. If the person who is ill is quietly listening to tapes, the person who is doing the care giving can relax and rest, too.

After an outing, whether a trip to the dentist or doctor, to the local market, or to visit a friend, plan a quiet time immediately upon returning home. Allow the individual time to rest before beginning a new activity. To minimize fatigue, avoid crowds and noisy, confusing places, bright, flickering lights, and loud music.

Always listen carefully and speak clearly and directly, especially when if an individual is tired. Fatigue raises the frustration level. Fatigue begets erratic behavior. Do all you can to avoid tiring an individual who has Alzheimer's disease.

Wandering

People with Alzheimer's disease are known for wandering off and getting lost. They are eager to go outside alone, and keeping them safe inside is a challenge. Telling an individual, "Don't go outside," or

"No, you can't go outside now," is a waste of time. Instead, try saying, "Fine, but let's have a cookie first." Often the person will have forgotten about asking to go outside. The request to go outside may arise again soon. When it does, find another diversion. "Come with me to get a piece of candy." "Let's look at this book." "Would you like to..." whatever you can think of at the time. Remember, diversion is the key. When individuals with Alzheimer disease are told "No," or "You can't," or "Don't do that," they more often than not become hostile and angry.

Try placing locks either high or low on the door. You are dealing with someone who has lost the ability to solve problems and rarely explores solutions outside the range of familiarity. A child-proof lock can also be installed.

Make sure the individual has an ID bracelet inscribed with the name, social security number, address and phone number. Be sure to include the area code. Register the patient with local law enforcement. Let neighbors know about the person's habit of walking off and ask for their cooperation.

Remember that the individual will get into a vehicle with anyone. If the individual still drives a car, driving off to nowhere in particular is a problem. The victim may go into stores and shoplift merchandise and become unruly and disorderly when confronted. An ID bracelet is essential in helping people contact the caregiver to come retrieve the person needing help.

Wanting To Go Home

One of the most common requests caregivers hear is, "I want to go home." This often comes from individuals in care facilities, but victims of Alzheimer's disease who are living in homes they have lived in for years also ask to go home. Maybe they are wanting to go home to their childhood homes, which is usually an impossibility. Home is where they find comfort and security, and comfort and security are difficult to find for someone whose mind and actions are out of control. The caregiver's head may well understand this, but for the caregiver's heart, it is a gut-wrenching request.

Caregivers feel guilty because their loved one is in a care facility in the first place instead of at home. They blame themselves for not taking their loved one home where he wants to be. Try explaining that they will go home later. The individual will not remember. Try not to feel personally torn. Know that the request will be made again and again just as a tired, little child asks repeatedly to go home. Say that it's okay. Say that we'll go home in a little while. Then distract them. Offer them something special, a snack, an activity, a walk outside, a TV program. It is futile to argue. Don't try to explain why they can't go home.

Loss of Hearing and Speech

Hearing loss is common in older people, but with those who have Alzheimer's disease, the loss is compounded. They have difficulty processing the information they can hear. They may hear only what makes sense to them at the time. They may hear part of the sentence and understand exactly the opposite of what was said. Speak clearly and directly to the individual, making sure you have made eye contact.

As the person loses ability to speak, frustration mounts. Often the frustration is expressed by swearing. Sentences are garbled. Using childhood expressions which have no meaning to anyone who didn't know the patient as a child is common. One person kept repeating, "Big dump. Big dump." The individual needed to use the bathroom and was using an expression from early childhood. No one in the room had the slightest idea of what the person meant until it was too late. Who would have guessed that "big dump" was the word for bowel movement?

Coping with Incontinence

Incontinence is common among victims of Alzheimer's disease and is one of the most difficult problems for the caregiver to deal with. If incontinence starts all of a sudden, find out if there is a cause that can be controlled. Is the individual on a new medication? Does the person have a bladder infection? Tranquilizers can make a person less sensitive to the urge to use the bathroom. If a check with the doctor shows no cause other than the disease, there are some things you can do that might help.

First, take the individual to the bathroom on a regular basis, either every hour or every two hours. This often helps. Make sure the person remembers where to find the toilet. Put a picture of a toilet or bathroom on the door. Some older people will recognize an outhouse as a bathroom, and that picture should go on the door, too. Many times when the individuals use the waste basket or the floor in the corner of the room, or the sink in the kitchen, or the grass outside, they have forgotten where the bathroom is or maybe even what it is for.

People with Alzheimer's disease have been known to see their reflections in the bathroom mirror and not recognize themselves. They might think that someone is in the bathroom watching them, and they are embarrassed. Try covering or removing the mirror.

Make sure that the person can remove clothing easily. Clothes that are difficult to get off and on make it difficult or even impossible for a person to use the bathroom. Elastic-waist, pull-down pants are easy to use and are commonly worn by both men and women.

Pads may cause victims to think they are in diapers and do not need to use the toilet. Sometimes cutting a hole in padding for men will make it easier for them to urinate while still protecting them from soiling themselves.

Some people with Alzheimer's disease will have forgotten what the toilet is for and will need to be shown repeatedly. Removing waste baskets can sometimes lessen a person's confusion.

One nursing home had placed a circle of black tiles at doorways to mark off-limits areas. When the Alzheimer's victims came to that black area, they would stop, thinking it was a hole in the ground. The black areas were working very well until two brothers, both former farmers, were admitted. These two made quite a splash. These brothers would urinate on the black tiles. The staff was quite upset and tired of cleaning up. Trying to figure out the problem, Johnny finally pointed out that when these men were young and plowing the fields and they had to relieve themselves, they probably wouldn't return to the house. They would most certainly go behind the tractor or a bush or a tree or even find a hole in the ground. Here in the care facility, they had found a convenient hole in the ground! As soon as the dark tiles were removed, the problem stopped.

A friend was traveling with her husband and they were waiting in the air terminal for their flight. For a brief time while she was not watching, her husband walked over to a potted palm tree and, oblivious to everyone, nonchalantly relieved himself. She was terribly embarrassed. It didn't bother him at all. He felt much better.

Accidents happen. Never, never scold or punish someone for having an accident. Although it is difficult when you are dealing with an adult who has just soiled their clothing or had an accident on the carpet, do remember to respect them and treat them with dignity. It is extremely important that you do. The individual has no control. The person doesn't want to make the caregiver angry. Those who have Alzheimer's disease are doing all they can possibly do to please the caregiver. Treat this helpless person with kindness. Alzheimer's victims need love just like the rest of us do. People need the same loving care at the end of their lives that they needed as babies in the beginning of their lives.

Trauma

When individuals with Alzheimer's disease have suffered a trauma, they most always deteriorate rapidly. Behavioral symptoms escalate. What can be an ordinary, every day experience to us can be traumatic to an Alzheimer's victim. Something as simple as rearranging the furniture can be upsetting. A trip to where there are crowds and confusion can be traumatic. An accident, a fall, an illness, surgery, all can cause a severe downturn. A spouse may die or divorce the victim. Any family crisis can trigger rapid deterioration. Victim's of Alzheimer's disease need routine, but life doesn't always cooperate. When traumas occur, expect a change.

Activities for the People with Alzheimer's Disease

Activities help structure time and bring a sense of normalcy to a person's day. Safe, meaningful activities can help maximize an individual's existing abilities. Activities that hold an individual's attention or keep a person occupied are a blessing to the caregiver as well.

Some activities will work for you and others will not. Don't be discouraged. Use the activities that work again and again. A person with Alzheimer's disease will not remember that he separated the green and red pasta shells yesterday. Be flexible. When an activity no longer works, discard it and try something else. You might try again on some of the ones that didn't work the first time.

Activities can allow the caregiver to enjoy time spent with the Alzheimer's victim, who is often the caregiver's spouse. Times of enjoying each other's company become more rare as the disease progresses. Activities can reduce agitation. They can be used to distract the individual from unacceptable behavior. They can ease the load carried by the caregiver.

We have included a few activities you may want to try. There are many. It is important to be creative. Adapt ideas to fit your needs. I strongly recommend that you look for books describing activities for individuals who have Alzheimer's disease. There are several that are filled with excellent ideas.

Walking

Daily exercise is an enjoyable and healthy activity. Individuals can walk alone if they know the route to take and do not wander. Walking provides a pleasant outing for caregiver and victim, if the victim can no longer walk alone.

For those in a care facility, walking alone is all right if there is a safe, enclosed area with well defined, continuous pathways. Individuals are confused if they come to "cross roads" where they must make a decision about which way to go. They will often stand helplessly at the intersection and wait for help.

Group walks with staff supervision are a good solution. Individuals have the advantage of social interaction. A more able person can assist a less able one by pushing a wheelchair or holding an elbow to steady a wobbly walking companion.

Dancing, Bowling and other Activities

For those who enjoyed dancing in their youth and still enjoy music and rhythm, dancing can be a fun, healthy exercise. Although the polka is a favorite, slow dancing is also very popular. People confined to a chair can sway their arms to the rhythm of the music.

Sometimes individual with Alzheimer's disease can still golf or bowl or even play tennis, but they can no longer keep score. How important is the score anyway? Names of fellow players will be forgotten. That doesn't matter either. What does matter is the enjoyment of the game. As long as individuals can maintain a physical activity or hobby, it is important that they have the opportunity to do so.

Helping with Household Chores

An individual can help set the table or do simple dinner preparations. Clean up is another area where an individual can help. Taking dishes from the table to the sink, or limit the task to clearing the silverware if that is all the person can handle. Folding towels and napkins is a good activity. Matching socks is another.

Give one task at a time. Appreciate the work done. Don't expect miracles. Help from someone suffering from Alzheimer's disease is often more work than no help at all, but it is important for the victim to contribute and feel valued. When your helper sets the table, don't worry if the fork ends up on the wrong side of the plate, or if the napkin folds are especially "creative." Relax if you possibly can. And remember, the order of the day is to praise and appreciate.

Sorting

Sort colored macaroni or pasta shells into different piles. Explain that you need help. This is not the time for you to play "quality control expert." Who cares if some reds are mixed in with the greens, or if the yellows aren't sorted out at all? This is an important job. Appreciate the help you are getting. People need to feel valued. They need to know that they are doing a good job. They need approval. Give it generously.

Think of other things that need sorting. Nuts of different shapes can be sorted. Brazil nuts and walnuts make a good selection. Have the individual put the Brazil nuts in one bowl and the walnuts in another. Try "napkin-sized" pieces of cloth. White napkins go in one basket. Green ones go in another. Sort playing cards. If the patient is able, sorting by suit can keep them busy. If you need to simplify card sorting, have them put all hearts in one stack, or all face cards in a stack. The choices are many. Be creative.

Do not use small items, such as small nuts, marbles, or buttons, that can be easily put into the mouth. There is a period of time when everything finds its way into the mouth. A marble can be seen as a grape. A button can be mistaken for a piece of candy. Not only can they ingest toxic material, individuals can choke on small items. Know and be ready to use the Heimlich maneuver. Use common sense. Always think of the individual's safety.

Art and Crafts

Art can be an excellent vehicle for reminiscing. Provide paints, brushes, and large sheets of paper. Remember that abstract art is beautiful. Be sure all paint is non-toxic. Individuals can tell about their drawings or paintings, providing the caregiver with insight into the person's past.

Cut and paste is a good activity. Make sure scissors do not have extremely sharp points. Neatness isn't a priority. Praise is. String large wooden beads. Stitch around pre-punched sewing cards using bright colored yarn and a large needle.

Recreate simplified versions of favorite games. Instead of playing volleyball with a ball, use a balloon. See how long a "team" can keep it in the air. When the balloon breaks, retrieve it immediately. Broken balloons are dangerous if swallowed. Be sure that balloon activity is supervised.

The Activity Apron

This apron or smock is a tried and true standby. The apron can be purchased, or if you are handy with a sewing machine, you can make one. Making an apron allows you to personalize it. Perhaps the recipient has a favorite color or loves brass buttons. Cover it with large buttons, appliqués attached to Velcro, pockets, zippers, bells that ring, a buckle on short "belt" that can be buckled and unbuckled, cords that can be braided, ribbons that can be tied into bows, or yarn tassels that can be fiddled with. Be creative. Have fun making the apron.

The Gadget Box

Fill a sturdy box with a variety of items, making sure that none have sharp edges. Pick up things from garage sales or the local thrift shop. Vary the texture and size. Include a coin purse that can be opened and then snapped shut, a pocket mirror, a string of beads, a feather, a soft toy. The choices are endless.

Miscellaneous Activity Ideas

Check out a "talking book" from the local library. Record your own voice reading one of your loved one's favorites. Reading the Bible on tape can provide hours of comfort. It also means that you can read it once, and an individual can hear it over and over, giving the caregiver some much needed, free time.

Train sets are popular. Lay the track in a figure eight and secure it to a board or table. Larger trains are easier to handle. The train should include an engine, a caboose, and several cars. Individuals enjoy arranging a station house, a farm house, and perhaps a few trees.

Music

Background music should not include vocals. Alzheimer's victims will try to find the person who is singing. Usually, music should be soft and soothing. Polka music is an exception. The polka was common fifty years ago and is another popular choice. Forget rock and roll! We all enjoy songs of our youth. Alzheimer's victims are no exception. Barbershop quartets and hymns are popular. Individuals will sing along with a record or with the group, especially if the song is a popular favorite. Have tapes and earphones available for individual listening.

Your attitude toward activities is as important as the activities. Approach each activity in a spirit of fun and joy. Your feelings are contagious. Keep your sense of humor. Laughter helps you to keep things in perspective, but laugh at your own mistakes. Never laugh at anyone else. Providing activities will help pass the time and ease the tension.

Placement: The Most Painful and Difficult Decision

When Johnny and I meet with a family who has found that one of their own has Alzheimer's disease, one of the first things we deal with is the possibility of placing their loved one in a nursing home. Even though the decision may be years away, prepare now. When the time comes, you will be ready.

One Step at a Time

One way to ease the process is to make the change in steps. We call it a transition time. Begin by taking the patient to an adult, day-care center. The staff is trained to manage the behavior of Alzheimer's patients and to provide safe and meaningful activities for them. By taking advantage of day care, the caregiver also is able to have a much needed break.

After an individual's regular visits to day care, we suggest a short-term placement of from three days to two weeks. Seeing that someone else is able to provide loving care can be reassuring to the caregiver. A short-term placement gives the caregiver a break, a little time, even if only a week or so, to live a reasonably normal life. Short-term placement helps a person realize that it is almost impossible for a single individual to give quality care twenty-four hours a day, seven days a week.

One of the most common complaints we hear is that the Alzheimer's victim won't go. They won't let caregivers out of sight. With persistence, just as you did when your young child didn't want to go to school, take the individual back again and again. At first, stay for a short period. Usually, they are quite content once they are there, and often will not want to leave when it comes time to go home.

A sad reality of Alzheimer's disease is that almost forty per cent of the caregivers die before the Alzheimer's victim. Providing care to someone with Alzheimer's disease is an exhausting job. Hours are long and difficult. There is no time off for good behavior. The emotional wear and tear is intense. We tell people over and over that there comes a time when one person can no longer do the job. We want to prepare families by helping them not to feel guilty, even though we know that almost everyone who places a loved one in a care facility feels guilty.

Carl had taken care of his wife Beth for several years and had coped quite successfully. One morning he called Johnny. Frustrated and discouraged, he needed help. It seemed that Carl could not get his wife out of bed. He had to carry her to the bathroom. He served her meals to her in bed on a tray. After the two men had shared a cup of coffee and conversation about the problems he was having with Beth, Carl asked if

Johnny would talk with her. They went into the bedroom where Beth was resting.

The first thing Johnny told her was that she looked very pretty. They talked a bit more, mostly Johnny telling her about how attractive she was. Then Carl and Johnny returned to the kitchen.

The next thing they knew, here came Beth walking down the hall. Johnny smiled at her and asked her if she was married. She promptly said she was not. Now, Beth and Carl had been married for over fifty years. When Johnny asked her for a date, she agreed to go immediately.

Johnny wasn't there to date Beth. He wanted to show Carl that different approaches sometimes worked, and that one person couldn't possibly have all of the answers all of the time. Sometimes it helps to let others with experience in dealing with people who suffer from Alzheimer's disease come up with new approaches and new solutions. It is easy to become bogged down under the strain of caring for someone all the time and all alone.

Beth had regressed to her teenage years where was she was being a typical teenager, difficult and rebellious. She would neither get out of bed nor cooperate in any other way.

Johnny and Carl laugh often about that visit, but the incident made it easier for Carl to make the decision he had been dreading for a long time. He began taking Beth to short-term day care on a regular basis. He told her he was taking her out on a date.

Carl had refused to even discuss permanent placement, but Beth's behavior was deteriorating in a hurry. The subject of long-term care is discussed frequently in support groups, and Carl was finally ready to listen. Nobody in the group condemned him for what he was now considering. Many had gone through the same thing. He began talking to his daughter about the possibility of placement. It took a while, but she was finally supportive. Within a year, Beth was placed in a care facility.

Caregivers need assurance from family members and close friends that it is okay to place a loved one who has Alzheimer's disease in a long-term care facility. They need someone to say, "Dad, it's okay to put Mom in a nursing home. We understand, and we think you're doing the right thing." Reassurance is very important.

Finding a Long-Term Care Facility: What To Look For

Learn what to look for in a facility. Understanding the needs of an individual with Alzheimer's disease is the first step in locating a home that provides quality care. They can't make decisions. It is the caretaker's job to decide for them.

Visit nursing homes in your area. Look for a facility that specializes in the care of people with Alzheimer's disease. Ask about the staff's training and experience. Observe the staff interacting with victims. Are they patient? Do they move and speak slowly? Do they use calm, modulated speech? Do they look individuals in the eye when speaking to them? Do they listen even when the person makes no sense? Are they courteous?

Are the surroundings clean and simple? People with Alzheimer's disease do not do well with confusion. Established routines and orderly, peaceful surroundings are a must. Soft, subtle colors are preferable. Walls should be plain, without design or ornamentation.

Does the facility smell fresh? Many places smell of urine, indicating lack of cleanliness and care. Avoid places with carpet in the resident areas. Accidents with those who have Alzheimer's disease are common, and it is almost impossible to remove the smell of urine from carpets.

Is the place uncluttered? It may appear sparse, but clutter can be confusing. Are patients dressed adequately or appropriately for the weather? Does the staff speak a language the patient can understand? If most of the residents speak English, does the staff speak English? If a person speaks only Spanish, is there a staff person who can speak Spanish with that person? Are there activities available that are led by a staff person?

Is there a safe yard where individuals are able to walk outside unattended? Are exit doors leading off the premises secured? Is the layout of pathways conducive to exercise? We recently visited a facility where individuals congregated at the point where the walkway intersected another in a "T" fashion. They had become confused and could not decide whether to go left or right or back the way they had come. Avoid situations where Alzheimer's victims are faced with having to make a decision. Look for continuous walkways. Figure eight designs work well. When paths wind in circular patterns without corners, individuals can walk without having to decide which way to go.

Are there any pets for the people to enjoy? Pets give abundant, unconditional love. One word from the patient brings the wag of a tail or the lick on the cheek. Pets provide adoration and acceptance people need. Especially people who are afflicted with Alzheimer's disease. I have watched an elderly woman stroke a purring cat for hours.

Are the floors plain or are they made of different colored squares so popular now, the ones that feature a black square and then a white square? The person with Alzheimer's disease confuses the dark squares with holes and walks carefully to avoid falling in. Sometimes the individual is afraid to walk on those checkered floors at all.

Does the dining room have square tables? Individuals want to find their same seat day after day. Round tables make it more difficult for them to locate their regular place. The dinnerware should be plain. Are healthy finger foods available? Snacks can help supply adequate nourishment.

What activities are there? Pat Warner has been a major contributor to our knowledge of good patient care. Her ideas and suggestions appear throughout this book. Each morning she provides a "job" for patients. A large jar of colored pasta is poured out onto a table. Individuals are told to put the red ones in one bowl, the plain ones in another bowl, and the green ones in yet another bowl. They busy themselves helping the cook prepare dinner. Everyone can relax and enjoy the job. A few green pastas mixed with the red ones is not going to spoil the soup. These pastas don't go into the soup anyway. Every day they do the same job.

Individuals can be involved in helping provide the necessities of their own care. They can fold clothes, dust, sweep, or set the table. Helping gives a sense of accomplishment. Expectations should be realistic. The duster will miss some spots. Clothes will not be folded perfectly. Sweeping is sometimes haphazard. The forks may be on the wrong side of the plate. A professional, caring staff person will give praise for work well done.

Visit the home. Spend some time. Walk around the grounds. Talk with the staff. Observe the people there. Observe how frequently restraints are used. Restraints can lead to anxiety, and anxiety can lead to more volatile behavior. There are times when restraints are necessary, either to protect the individual or to protect others from the individual. Alternative solutions should be explored before restraints are used. Ask the staff about individuals who are restrained and discuss the facility's philosophy and approach toward using restraints.

Johnny recently received a video produced by a major university on what to look for in choosing a care facility. He uses that video to show all the things you shouldn't do. They recommend that a flower be placed by each resident's room. Anyone working in an Alzheimer's facility will tell you that the Alzheimer's patient will think the flower is finger food and try to eat it. Forget the flowers. Remember the hugs.

The most important thing, more important than anything I have mentioned so far, is how you feel about the people running the facility. Are they gentle and caring? Are you comfortable leaving your loved one with them? Placement is difficult at best. Caretakers are tormented with guilt when they have to leave a loved one in a place where the quality of care is in question.

Facilities are improving. Good ones are available. When the time comes to make the decision, you will be more comfortable if you are familiar with the choices available in selecting a nursing home. It is worth the time and trouble it takes to find the right one.

Clothing and Personal Items Needed in a Care Facility

What to take? What to leave? At a time when the caregiver is making one of the most difficult decisions of a lifetime, placing a loved one in a long-term care facility, you have to pack. The nuts and bolts of packing must be attended to. The individual facility may have specific requests. Hopefully, this list of the basics might help. Again, our warmest thanks to Pat Warner.

Personal Items

These must include personal hygiene items:
tooth brush and paste
hair brush and comb
razor or electric shaver
shaving cream
lotions, cologne, cosmetics if used
nail file, nail clippers

Other personal items may include:
Bible
favorite blanket or pillow
favorite afghan or shawl
any small, favorite item loved by the
victim
old-time family photos

Don't send too many things. When selecting photographs, choose those taken long ago. Recent photos are often not recognized, since the patient in a care facility is usually in the latter stages of the disease and is living sometime in the past. Include pictures of the wife or husband when they were young or the now-grown children when they were young children. A picture of a favorite childhood pet is often appreciated.

Remember that it is the family's responsibility to mark all belongings with the individual's name. Permanent labels can be purchased and sewn securely on cloth items. Identify the photos on their reverse side. Check items frequently to be sure they are in good repair and marked.

Clothing

The key is to select clothing that is easy to care for, easy to get on and off, and nonrestrictive. Avoid zippers and buttons if possible. No dry cleaning items, please. It is the family's responsibility to keep clothing in good repair and replaced as needed. Be sure to provide a change of clothes for the change of seasons.

A Sample List

Clothing for Men and Women

7 changes of underclothing
1 pair dress shoes
1 robe
1 light jacket
5 handkerchiefs
5 sweat pants
3 nightshirts, night gowns or pajamas
1 or 2 cardigan sweaters
1 pair washable slippers, Velcro preferred
2 pair washable sneakers
10 pair white cotton socks. (No other colors)

For Men
3 pairs trousers
(suspenders optional)
2 dress shirts

For Women
5 dresses or slacks

3 blouses for
slacks

1 belt for pants	3 bras
2 pair dress socks	3 pair pantyhose/ knee-highs

Now that you are packed and ready, there is another important task to be done. To give a person with Alzheimer's disease the best possible care, it is important to give the staff at the facility as much information on your loved one as you possibly can.

A Sample Personal Profile

Alzheimer's disease takes a person on journey back through that person's life. Caregivers struggle to find ways to help the individual along this rocky and treacherous road. Knowing the person's history is helpful.

This sample personal profile, developed by Pat Warner of Oregon, is designed to help you gather and organize pertinent information. Many caregivers are spouses who married the Alzheimer's victim later in life when first marriages had ended and children had grown. Some did not know the victim as a young man or woman, and may need to talk with friends and relatives who knew the individual as a child or young adult in order to find as much information as possible.

Gather all the information you can. Something is better than nothing. Don't worry if you are unable to provide information to all of the requests below. This is not a test. It is a tool to assist you. If you have helpful information that is not requested, be sure to add it.

The more that is known about a patient, the better. You are welcome to use any of this material in any way you might find useful. Copy the information, and if there is not enough room on the survey for you to write what you need to write, use additional sheets of paper. Examples are given to show how information can be presented, however, there are no right or wrong ways. Whatever you put down will be appreciated.

General Information:

Name of Alzheimer's Victim:
Nick name(s) or pet name(s):
Caregivers name:
Current Address of Caregiver:
Phone:

List the addresses or places the patient lived as a child:

List the city, state, or country where the patient lived as a child. Example: A small town in Texas. New York City. The Philippines. If patient moved often, list other places lived.

Language(s) Spoken in the Patient's Childhood Home:

As the patient reverts to a childhood language, it is helpful for the staff to find someone who speaks that language and communicate with the patient.

Work History:

List previous occupations and/or professions. Examples: pilot, artist, farmer, painter, lawyer, business person, teacher, or doctor. Give as much detail as you can. High school math teacher or kindergarten teacher. Surgeon, general practitioner, or psychiatrist? Did the patient change jobs often? Truck driver, carpenter, salesman.

Patient's Childhood:

Briefly describe patient's early years.

Example One: Man/rancher. Patient grew up on cattle ranch in eastern Texas. He is the third born in a family of seven children, four boys and three girls. He is the second son. Enjoyed riding, fishing, hunting, camping. Active in 4H activities. Competed in calf-roping contests in local rodeos.

Example Two: Woman/dancer. Patient grew up in New York City. Only child. Father was a surgeon. Mother was an artist. Attended private schools. Patient loved theater and the arts. Studied ballet, starting at an early age. Quiet child. Loved her Persian cat named Fluff. Closest friend was her first cousin, Carolyn, nicknamed Kiko. Loved to read, especially poetry.

Patient's Young Adulthood:

Single or married; how many times and duration of each marriage. List names of all spouses. Patient may think former spouse is the current spouse. Number of children. Health problems in family. Community, school, and church activities. Hobbies.

Example One: Man/Rancher. Patient married at twenty-one to high school sweetheart. He worked first as a ranch hand, and then bought his own place. They had three children, two boys and a girl. Oldest son had polio. Wife killed in auto accident when she was twenty-six. Patient remarried. Second marriage didn't last. No children from second marriage. Married again. Third wife was a widow with four children. Raised step children as his own. Family active in Methodist church. Wife loved to garden. He continued his interest in rodeo. All kids active in 4H.

Example Two: Woman/dancer. Professional ballerina. Injured in fall. Had to give up dancing. Married man much older than she. Had no children. Widowed at age forty-five. Never remarried. Always had cats. Loved cats. Became a recluse, but continued to see her cousin Kiko. Lived in the past, surrounded by memorabilia of her dancing career.

Late Adulthood - Retirement Years:

Retirement activities. Did the patient move? Was patient active in service clubs, community, church, etc. List leisure activities.

Example One: Man/rancher. Sold ranch after children were grown. None wanted to continue ranching. Moved to retirement community in Florida. Had difficulty adjusting to new life. Missed ranch in Texas. Always wanted to return. Was planning to move back when signs of illness began. He and his wife became close friends with Clarence and Hazel. Took up golf. Wife active in garden club. Both play bridge.

Example Two: Woman/dancer. Lived alone with cats. Read constantly until no longer able to. Symptoms of disease began in her late fifties. Few friends. Sees cousin Kiko, who visits regularly. Remembers names of other dancers, Karen and Marianne. Unable to care for herself.

Family:

List names and relationship to patient. Include: wife (wives) husband(s), brothers, sisters, parents, children, grandparents, uncles, aunts, cousins, etc.

Name:
Relationship:

Friends:

Example: Mike: golfing buddy. Sam: best friend as boys. Jean: neighbor. Kiko: cousin.

Name:
When:

Pets:

List kind of animal: dog, cat, horse, parakeet. Why special?

Pet
Name
Why Special?

Examples: Dog, black mongrel, Midnight, constant companion. Horse, gelding, Big Red, ridden in rodeo competition. Persian cat, Fluff, childhood pet.

Favorite Activities:

Examples: TV, radio, reading, sewing, knitting, hunting, fishing, camping, travel, sports, watching sports on TV, exercise, cards, golf, bowling, theater, painting, church activities, square dancing.

Personal Care Needs:

Note specific information unique to this patient, such as food sensitivities or allergies, eating, bathing, toilet habits, sleep patterns, medications, glasses, hearing aids, dentures, cane or walker.

Spiritual Needs:

List religious preference and any specific religious practices that would enhance the patient's stay in the care facility. Example: Gospel singing, Bible reading, prayer groups, visitation from priest or pastor.

Other Comments:

Are there special problems and/or concerns not addressed in this profile sheet? For example: racial or sexual prejudice, phobias, obsessions, or needs for attention. Are there any special talents, such as the ability to play an instrument or sing?

Summary

Those with Alzheimer's disease come from all walks of life, all races and religions, all educational levels. Alzheimer's disease is an equal opportunity killer. Each individual brings a unique personality and personal history. The disease affects each differently.

Although victims of Alzheimer's disease often act like children, never treat them as though they were children. Never patronize an individual who is sick. Never talk in front of them as though they were not there. Respect each individual's dignity. The Alzheimer's victim's sense of security and acceptance is paramount. Love, kindness, and reassurance help build and maintain that secure sense.

Be creative. Never be harsh. Agree with the victim. Never argue. Never try to explain. Distract them. Divert their attention to something else. Wait a few minutes and try again.

We offer these suggestions knowing that there are no pat answers, no guaranteed solutions. We hope some of these suggestions have been helpful to you.

INDEX   BOOK TWO

ORDER FORM

for

WILL I BE NEXT?

Name _____

Address _____

City/State/Zip _____

Phone _____

Send check for $14.00 ($12.00 for book and $2 for shipping/ handling). California orders add 7.75 % sales tax.

HopeWarren Press
P.O. Box 204
Acampo, CA 95220

Or phone 209-368-3662 for orders
or further information, including quantity discounts.